D1591855

ITI Treatment Guide
Volume 2

ITI
Treatment
Guide

Editors:
D. Wismeijer, D. Buser, U. Belser

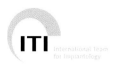

Authors:
D. Morton, J. Ganeles

Volume 2

Loading Protocols
in Implant Dentistry

Partially Dentate Patients

Quintessence Publishing Co, Ltd
Berlin, Chicago, London, Tokyo, Barcelona,
Beijing, Istanbul, Milan, Moscow, New Delhi,
Paris, Prague, São Paulo, Seoul, Warsaw

German National Library CIP Data

The German National Library has listed this publication in the German National Bibliography. Detailed bibliographical data are available on the Internet at http://dnb.ddb.de.

 © 2008 Quintessence Publishing Co, Ltd
Ifenpfad 2-4, 12107 Berlin,
www.quintessenz.de

Medical Editing: Dr. Kati Benthaus, CH-Basel
Illustrations: Ute Drewes, CH-Basel,
                     www.drewes.ch
Copyediting: Triacom Dental, D-Barendorf,
                     www.triacom-dental.de
Graphic Concept: Wirz Corporate AG, CH-Zurich
Production: Bernd Burkart, D-Berlin
Printing: Bosch-Druck GmbH, D-Landshut,
                     www.bosch-druck.de

Printed in Germany

ISBN: 978-3-938947-12-8

The components of the implant system shown are part of the Straumann® Dental Implant System.

The tooth identification system used in this ITI Treatment Guide is that of the FDI World Dental Federation.

The ITI Mission is ...

"... to promote and disseminate knowledge on all aspects of implant dentistry and related tissue regeneration through research, development and education to the benefit of the patient."

Preface

Implant dentistry is probably the most interesting and dynamic discipline in modern dental science. It has evolved from a trial-and-error field to an evidence-based predictable treatment modality. This has given dentistry a whole new palette of options for patient treatment. The loading protocols advocated in the early years of implant dentistry (3 to 6 months) are now behind us. Due to advances in surgical and prosthetic protocols as well as the innovation of implant surfaces, the conventional healing period before loading has been brought down to 6 weeks or even less. According to the Proceedings of the Third ITI Consensus Conference, published in a special 2004 supplement of JOMI, immediate implant loading is defined as restoring the implant with a provisional or final restoration in occlusal contact within 24 hours. Immediate implant loading, properly carried out, has shortened the transitional period between implant placement and implant restoration immensely. This has many benefits for our patients when we look at total treatment time, the number of clinic visits, comfort during the healing period, and esthetic and phonetic aspects of the implant treatment. At the same conference, early loading was defined as the prosthetic loading or utilization of an implant at any time between immediate and conventional loading, and conventional loading was defined as the restoration and loading of an implant after a healing period of 3 to 6 months. These definitions are likely to be reviewed in the future, as today's evidence-based and improved techniques allow for shorter healing periods to be considered predictable and safe.

Immediate loading always includes an element of risk. As in the ITI Treatment Guide Volume 1, where each patient's esthetic risk profile was presented, in Volume 2 we have chosen to present a treatment risk profile for immediate loading, which will be a great help for clinicians planning cases that involve choices between various implant loading protocols. This risk profile instrument can be used as an indicator to predict the risk involved in not reaching an acceptable result when treating patients following an immediate loading concept. Optimal results in immediate implant loading can only be achieved when following a comprehensive clinical protocol based on science, preoperative diagnosis, treatment planning, and precise management of the patient treatment, and, last but not least, experience. Based on this, we have included the SAC (Straightforward, Advanced, and Complex) classification for all the patients presented in this volume. The SAC classification, which is based on a series of items that are checked for every patient, gives the dentist insight into the complexity of each individual patient. The SAC classification for implant dentistry, as described in this volume, will soon be published in book form, reflecting the results of a consensus conference organized by the ITI in March 2007.

Supported by the literature, the results of the ITI Consensus Conference, which were published in a special 2004 supplement of the JOMI, and a large variety of clinical cases, this second volume of the ITI Treatment Guide presents comprehensive details on how to treat patients with crowns and fixed dental prostheses on implants following immediate, early, and conventional loading protocols.

Daniel Wismeijer   Daniel Buser   Urs C. Belser

Acknowledgment

The authors wish to express their special thanks to Dr. Kati Benthaus for her excellent support and outstanding commitment to maintaining the high quality of this second in the series of ITI Treatment Guides.

Editors and Authors

Editors:

Urs C. Belser, DMD, Professor
   University of Geneva
   Department of Prosthodontics
   School of Dental Medicine
   Rue Barthélemy-Menn 19,1211 Genève 4, Switzerland
   E-mail: urs.belser@medecine.unige.ch

Daniel Buser, DMD, Professor
   University of Berne
   Department of Oral Surgery and Stomatology
   School of Dental Medicine
   Freiburgstrasse 7, 3010 Bern, Switzerland
   E-mail: daniel.buser@zmk.unibe.ch

Daniel Wismeijer, DMD, Professor
   Academic Center for Dentistry Amsterdam (ACTA)
   Free University
   Department of Oral Function
   Section of Implantology and Prosthetic Dentistry
   Louwesweg 1, 1066 EA Amsterdam, Netherlands
   E-mail: dwismeij@acta.nl

Authors:

Jeffrey Ganeles, DMD
   Florida Institute for Periodontics & Dental Implants
   3020 North Military Trail, Suite 200
   Boca Raton, FL 33431, USA
   Adjunct Associate Professor
   Nova Southeastern University College
   of Dental Medicine
   Ft. Lauderdale, FL 33328, USA
   E-mail: jganeles@perio-implant.com;

Dean Morton, BDS, MS
   University of Florida, Gainesville
   Center for Implant Dentistry
   Department of Oral and Maxillofacial Surgery
   1600 W Archer Road, D7-6, Gainesville, FL 32610, USA
   E-mail: dmorton@dental.ufl.edu

Contributors

Stephen Chen, MDSc, Dr
School of Dental Science
The University of Melbourne
720 Swanston Street
Melbourne, VIC 3010, Australia
E-mail: schen@balwynperio.com.au

Anthony Dickinson, BDSC, MSD
1564 Malvern Road
Glen Iris, VIC 3146, Australia
E-mail: ajd1@iprimus.com.au

Christopher Evans, BDSc Hons (Qld), MDSc (Melb)
75 Asling St., Brighton
Melbourne, VIC 3186, Australia
E-mail: cdjevans@mac.com

German O. Gallucci, DMD, Dr med dent
Assistant Professor
Harvard School of Dental Medicine
Department of Restorative Dentistry
and Biomaterial Sciences
188 Longwood Avenue, Boston, MA 02115, USA
E-mail: german_gallucci@hsdm.harvard.edu

Christopher Hart, BDSc, Grad Dip Clin Dent, MDSc
4 Linckens Cres
Balwyn, VIC 3103, Australia
E-mail: cnhart@mac.com

Frank Higginbottom, DDS
3600 Gaston Avenue, Suite 1107
Dallas, TX 75246, USA
E-mail: bottom@dallasesthetics.com

Murray Kaufman, DDS
9911 W. Pico Blvd., Suite 780
Los Angeles, CA 90035, USA
E-mail: murray300@aol.com

William C. Martin, DMD, MS
University of Florida, Gainesville
Center for Implant Dentistry
Department for Oral and Maxillofacial Surgery
1600 W Archer Road, D7-6
Gainesville, FL 32610, USA
E-mail: wmartin@dental.ufl.edu

Yasushi Nakajima, DDS
3-10-1 Higashihagoromo Takaishi
Osaka, 592-0003, Japan
E-mail: njdc3805@crest.ocn.ne.jp

Mario Roccuzzo, DMD, Dr med dent
Corso Tassoni 14, Torino, 10143, Italy
E-mail: mroccuzzo@iol.it

Adam Rosenberg, BDS, MS
401 Wattletree Rd
Malvern East, VIC 3145, Australia
E-mail: perio@bigpond.net.au

James Ruskin, DMD, MD, Professor
University of Florida, Gainesville
College of Dentistry
P.O. Box 100416, Gainesville, FL 32601, USA
E-mail: jruskin@dental.ufl.edu

Bruno Schmid, DMD
Bayweg 3, 3123 Belp, Switzerland
E-mail: brunoschmid@vtxmail.ch

Gary Solnit, DDS, MS
9675 Brighton Way, Suite 330
Beverly Hills, CA 90210, USA
E-mail: gssolnit@earthlink.net

Francesca Vailati, MD, DMD, MSc
Senior Lecturer
University of Geneva
Department of Prosthodontics
School of Dental Medicine
Rue Barthélemy-Menn 19
1211 Genève 4, Switzerland
E-mail: francesca.vailati@medecine.unige.ch

Thomas G. Wilson Jr, DDS, PA
Periodontics and Dental Implants
5465 Blair Road, Suite 200
Dallas, TX 75231, USA
E-mail: tom@tgwperio.com

Table of Contents

1   <u>Introduction</u>

D. Morton

Through research, development and education, the ITI has a mission to promote and disseminate knowledge on all aspects of implant dentistry and related tissue regeneration. Positioned at the forefront of a dynamic and exciting era in implant dentistry, the ITI has assumed, through its Education Committee and projects, a leading role in the delivery of information to the professional community and their patients.

Endeavors of particular relevance to this mission include:

- The ITI Consensus Conferences, which are held periodically to allow for the systematic and critical evaluation of existing knowledge as it relates to recent and perhaps controversial trends in implant dentistry.
- The ITI Treatment Guides, which provide readers with objective and simplified recommendations for patient treatment that are documented by science, supported by experienced clinicians, and beneficial to patients.

The ITI Treatment Guide Volume 2 is devoted to the restoration of partially dentate patients. Central to this volume of the ITI Treatment Guide are loading protocols available to the clinician and the patient, and how they relate to various treatment indications, including both single and multiple missing teeth in the posterior and anterior regions of the mouth.

Through the presentation of the findings from the ITI Consensus Conference held in 2003, historic reference and a range of patient treatments, it is anticipated that this volume of the ITI Treatment Guide will provide concise and meaningful recommendations that can improve the prospects of optimal treatment for patients. The authors believe that this volume will provide a valuable reference and resource that will help clinicians and patients achieve their treatment goals.

2 Proceedings of the Third ITI Consensus Conference: Loading Protocols in Implant Dentistry

With over 4500 Fellows and Members in more than 40 countries, the International Team for Implantology (ITI) is a non-profit academic organization of professionals in implant dentistry and tissue regeneration. The ITI organizes Consensus Conferences at 5-year intervals to discuss relevant topics in implant dentistry.

The first and second ITI Consensus Conferences in 1993 and 1998 (Proceedings of the ITI Consensus Conference, published in 2000) primarily discussed basic surgical and prosthetic issues in implant dentistry. The third ITI Consensus Conference was convened in 2003. For this conference, the ITI Education Committee decided to focus the discussion on four special topics that had received much attention in recent years, "Loading Protocols for Endosseous Dental Implants" being one of them (Proceedings of the Third ITI Consensus Conference, JOMI Special Supplement, 2004).

One group, under the leadership of Professor David Cochran, was asked to focus on, review the relevant literature on, and find consensus relating to loading protocols for endosseous dental implants.

Group participants:	Matteo Chiapasco
	Roberto Cornelini
	Kerstin Fischer
	Jeffrey Ganeles
	Siegfried Heckmann
	Robert A. Jaffin
	Regina Mericske-Stern
	Dean Morton
	Ates Parlar
	Edwin Rosenberg
	Paul Rousseau
	Yoshikazu Soejima
	Pedro Tortamano
	Wilfried Wagner
	Hans-Peter Weber
	Daniel Wismeijer

2.1 Consensus Statements and Recommended Clinical Procedures Regarding Loading Protocols for Endosseous Dental Implants

D. Morton

The group was asked to develop evidence-based reviews on topics related to various loading protocols for dental implants. The following literature reviews were prepared and presented to the group for discussion:

- Matteo Chiapasco: "Early and Immediate Restoration and Loading of Implants in Completely Edentulous Patients"

- Jeffrey Ganeles, Daniel Wismeijer: "Early and Immediately Restored and Loaded Dental Implants for Single-Tooth and Partial-Arch Applications"

- Dean Morton, Robert Jaffin, Hans-Peter Weber: "Immediate Restoration and Loading of Dental Implants: Clinical Considerations and Protocols"

The prime objective of the literature reviews was to determine whether a procedure could be recommended as routine based on the available evidence. The second objective was to identify whether patients perceived a benefit associated with these procedures.

At the ITI Consensus Conference, the authors presented their manuscripts to the group for discussion. There was discussion concerning how the authors approached writing the draft, how the literature was searched and reviewed, what the major findings were, and finally, what conclusions could be drawn.

During the discussion, several statements were made regarding immediate or early restoration and/or loading of implants in edentulous and partially dentate patients. These are listed below, along with issues that were identified throughout the discussions.

2.1.1 Definition of Terms

In recent years, confusion has been evident with terminology as it relates to loading protocols in implant dentistry. The group discussed this terminology in detail, in relation to both existing literature and ITI consensus. Most of these terms were defined in a conference on immediate and early loading that was held in Spain in May 2002 (Aparicio and coworkers, 2003). However, the group modified these definitions for use in their report. The modified definitions are presented here:

Conventional loading
The prosthesis is attached in a second procedure after a healing period of 3 to 6 months.

Early loading
A restoration in contact with the opposing dentition and placed at least 48 hours after implant placement but not later than 3 months afterward.

Immediate restoration
A restoration inserted within 48 hours of implant placement but not in occlusion with the opposing dentition.

Immediate loading
A restoration placed in occlusion with the opposing dentition within 48 hours of implant placement.

Delayed loading
The prosthesis is attached in a second procedure that takes place some time later than the conventional healing period of 3 to 6 months.

2.1.2   Review of Loading Protocols

The choice of loading protocols should be viewed as dependent, among other factors on two distinct processes: primary and secondary bone contact. By understanding these concepts, it is possible to appreciate how various loading protocols are viable and why they are dependent on these processes.

Primary bone contact
As soon as an implant is placed into the jawbone, certain areas of the implant surface are in direct contact with bone.

Secondary bone contact
As healing occurs, the bone around the implant surface is remodeled, and areas of new bone contact with the implant surface appear. This remodeled bone and new bone contact, termed secondary bone contact, predominates at later healing times when the amount of primary contact is decreased.

Shortened loading protocols
Immediate and early loading protocols should focus on (1) the amount of primary bone contact, (2) the quantity and quality of bone at the implant site, and (3) the rapidity of bone formation around the implant.

Immediate loading
When existing bone of high quality and quantity is found and when other factors are favorable, immediate loading of the implant may be possible.

Early loading
If the existing bone is not of high quality and quantity, then bone formation must occur within a relatively short time so that early loading of the implants can take place.

Direct occlusal contact
In the case of direct occlusal contact, the restoration makes contact with the opposing dentition.

Indirect occlusion
With indirect occlusion, the implant is restored without directly contacting the opposing dentition, i.e. it is out of occlusion.

Progressive loading
With progressive loading, the implant is restored in "light" contact initially and is gradually brought into full contact with the opposing dentition.

2.1.3 Consensus Statements

With the understanding that the literature base is small and the strength of evidence graded as inadequate to fair, the group reached the following conclusions with regard to loading protocols for endosseous dental implants in 2003:

Statements A:
Edentulous Mandible

Statements B:
Edentulous Maxilla

Statement A.1
In edentulous mandibles, the immediate loading of 4 implants with an overdenture in the interforaminal area with rigid bar fixation and cross-arch stabilization is a predictable and well-documented procedure.

Statement B.1
No articles were found supporting immediate or early loading of implants with an overdenture in the edentulous maxilla. Therefore, this procedure would have to be considered experimental at this time.

Statement A.2
The early loading of implants (splinted or unsplinted) in the edentulous mandible with an overdenture is not well-documented.

Statement B.2
In the edentulous maxilla, immediate or early loading of implants utilizing a fixed prosthesis is not well-documented.

Statement A.3
Immediate loading of implants supporting fixed restorations in the edentulous mandible is a predictable and well-documented procedure, provided that a relatively large number of implants are placed.

Statement A.4
The Consensus Group found only six publications supporting the early loading of implants in the edentulous mandible with a fixed restoration.

Statements C:
Partially Dentate Mandible or Maxilla

Statements D:
Other Issues Discussed

Statement C.1
In the partially dentate maxilla and mandible, the immediate restoration or loading of implants supporting fixed prostheses is not well-documented. It should be noted that in many of these cases the restoration is not in contact with the opposing dentition. This observation highlights the care that must be expended to plan and successfully complete such a restoration.

Statement C.2
The early restoration or loading of titanium implants with a roughened surface supporting fixed prostheses after 6 to 8 weeks of healing is well-documented and predictable in the partially dentate maxilla and mandible. Results seem to indicate that the outcome is similar to results obtained with conventional procedures. However, further studies are necessary before these procedures can be proposed as routine due to the limited number of implants placed in comparison to the number of conventionally loaded implants, and the short follow-up period.

Statement C.3
Interproximal crestal bone levels and soft tissue changes adjacent to immediately restored or loaded implants were found to be similar to those reported for conventional loading protocols.

Statement D.1
A conventional loading period of 3 to 6 months is likely to be modified for implants with roughened surfaces. The 3- to 6-month period was originally defined for implants with machined surfaces, and it is well-documented that the machined surface is not as successful as the roughened surface in certain indications.

Statement D.2
A question that needs to be addressed is whether the patient benefits from an immediate or early loading protocol. There is an associated risk with immediate and/or early loading, and this risk must be evaluated in terms of patient benefit. Postoperative care must be evaluated in such calculations.

Statement D.3
A related question is whether conventional loading is justified in certain cases. For example, does delaying the restoration of an implant place the patient at a disadvantage?

Statement D.4
The types of occlusal schemes need to be specified in various loading protocols. Occlusal schemes for immediately and early loaded implants that result in successful outcomes need to be determined.

2.1.4   Clinical Recommendations

The following types of treatment were recommended by the Consensus Group in 2003 (published in a supplement of JOMI in 2004), provided that all other aspects of diagnosis and treatment planning have been performed and are considered acceptable by the clinician. Immediate restoration and loading procedures are considered advanced or complex. As such, it is assumed that the clinician has the requisite level of skills and experience. The recommendations are based on the literature available in 2003 and the collective experience of the Consensus Working Group.

Immediate Restoration or Loading:

Edentulous mandible
Four implants are suitable for use in 2 protocols: an overdenture retained and/or supported by a bar that rigidly connects the implants, or a fixed restoration on a framework (acrylic resin and/or metal) that rigidly connects the implants. More than 4 implants are suited for rigid provisional restoration connecting all of the implants, or for a fixed restoration on a framework (acrylic resin and/or metal) that rigidly connects the implants.

Edentulous maxilla
No routine procedure is recommended.

Partially dentate maxilla and mandible
No routine procedure is recommended.

**Early Restoration or Loading:
Edentulous Mandible**

Two implants
Two implants may be placed to retain an overdenture, supported by a bar connecting the implants or by freestanding implants, when the implants are characterized by a rough titanium surface and allowed to heal for at least 6 weeks.

Four implants
In a four-implant scenario, either of two options is recommended: an overdenture retained and supported by a bar connecting the implants or by unconnected implants, or a fixed restoration on a framework that rigidly connects the implants. The implants should be characterized by a rough titanium surface and allowed to heal for at least 6 weeks.

More than four implants
More than four implants may be used for a fixed restoration on a framework that rigidly connects the implants; again, the implants are characterized by a rough titanium surface and allowed to heal for at least 6 weeks.

Edentulous Maxilla

Four different early loading scenarios are possible:

> **Four implants retaining an overdenture...**
> ...supported by a bar connecting the implants or by un-connected implants, with implants characterized by a rough titanium surface and allowed to heal for at least 6 weeks. The site must be characterized by type 1, 2 or 3 bone.

> **Four implants supporting a fixed restoration...**
> ...on a framework that rigidly connects the implants. As with the above scheme, the implants are characterized by a rough titanium surface and allowed to heal for at least 6 weeks, and the site is characterized by type 1, 2 or 3 bone.

> **More than four implants retaining an overdenture...**
> ...supported by a bar connecting the implants or by un-connected implants, with implants characterized by a rough titanium surface and allowed to heal for at least 6 weeks, in a site characterized by type 1, 2 or 3 bone.

> **More than four implants supporting a fixed restoration...**
> ...on a framework that rigidly connects the implants. Again, the implants are characterized by a rough tita-nium surface and allowed to heal for at least 6 weeks, and the site is characterized by type 1, 2 or 3 bone.

Partially Dentate Maxilla and Mandible

A fixed prosthesis is recommended in these cases:

> **Implant number and distribution are dependent on patient circumstances...**
> ...including bone quality and quantity, number of miss-ing teeth, condition of opposing dentition, type of oc-clusion, and bruxism. Implants must be characterized by a rough titanium surface and are allowed to heal for at least 6 weeks and in type 1, 2 or 3 bone.

2.1.5   Conclusions

The Third ITI Consensus Conference took place in August 2003. The Consensus Statements phrased by Working Group 3, exploring the topic of "Loading Protocols for En-dosseous Dental Implants," were based on the body of lit-erature available at that time. It is recognized that, in 2003, many of the clinical recommendations suggested by the Consensus Group were not yet associated with strong evidence. Readers should note that the experience of the group was used in formulating the recommendations.

Meanwhile, the topic of loading protocols for endosseous implants has been further researched, and additional lit-erature was published. In addition, new surface technolo-gies and their influence on immediate and early loading protocols, were investigated.

Chapter 2.2, entitled "Review of Implant Loading Proto-cols," recognizes the evolution of implant loading proto-cols, including recent data and literature, in order to give a state-of-the-art overview of implant loading protocols in connection with the clinical implications and applications to be derived from them.

2.2 Review of Implant Loading Protocols

J. Ganeles

2.2.1 Original Loading Protocols

Osseointegration became recognized as a stable, predictable and desirable biological interface in implant dentistry through careful documentation originally credited to Brånemark (Brånemark and coworkers, 1977; Albrektsson, 1983; Albrektsson, 1995) and to Schroeder and coworkers (1976). These authors demonstrated enhanced predictability and longevity associated with this ankylotic bone-to-implant condition. Previous concepts, as described by Linkow and coworkers (1977), who advocated the establishment of a fibrous tissue layer surrounding the implant to simulate the periodontal ligament, were not predictable (Smithloff and Fritz, 1976; Smithloff and Fritz, 1987).

The early publications on osseointegration (Albrektsson and coworkers, 1981) suggested principles and techniques to predictably achieve this result. Both Brånemark and Schroeder identified the need for minimally traumatic, precise osteotomy preparation, sterile technique, suitable biomaterials, and unloaded or stress-free healing. Brånemark's protocol required submucosal healing for 3 to 6 months, depending on anatomical location, while Schroeder's permitted trans-mucosal healing for 3 to 4 months. Ultimately, these intervals were acknowledged to be empirical in nature (Brånemark and coworkers, 1985; Brånemark, 2001).

In a review article by Szmukler-Moncler and coworkers (2000), various explanations for the long, delayed healing periods recommended by early authors were considered. They suggested that in preliminary treatment trials, factors such as patients with poor bone quality, non-optimized implant design or surfaces, non-optimized surgical protocols, and non-optimized prosthetic treatment protocols were included. In the transitional 1980s, when the predictability of osseointegrated dental implants was widely questioned, healing protocols were advocated to overcompensate for these negative factors. Since earlier developers and authors were struggling to convince the professional community that implants should be considered "lege artis" in dentistry (Brånemark and coworkers, 1977), long, stress-free healing periods were recommended.

Research regarding wound healing of the bone-implant interface has shown that several factors are important in order to establish osseointegration. Early work in orthopedics

by Cameron and coworkers (1973), Schatzker and coworkers (1975), Søballe and coworkers (1992) and others became known to researchers in implant dentistry, showing the importance of surface texture and biomechanical stability during the early healing phase. This information was further reviewed and reinforced with respect to implant dentistry by Szmukler-Moncler and coworkers (1998). Earlier observations by Brunski and coworkers (1979), Deporter and coworkers (1986), Akagawa and coworkers (1986), Khang and coworkers (2001), and others highlighted the importance of implant texture, shape, and biomechanical stability in terms of contributing to healing outcomes.

Summarizing the knowledge obtained through research and clinical observations, it can be stated that for a dental implant to achieve osseointegration, several factors are important. These include:

- The placement of an implant composed of or coated with a suitable biocompatible material, such as titanium, tantalum, hydroxylapatite, zirconia (Kohal and coworkers, 2006), gold alloy (Abrahamsson and Cardaropoli, 2007), or others.
- Site preparation without excessive thermal, traumatic, bacterial, or biological injury to the host bed.
- The adequate stabilization of the implant (Lioubavina-Hack and coworkers, 2006) to eliminate movement below the threshold of deleterious micromovement, estimated to be 50 – 150 microns (Szmukler-Moncler and coworkers, 1998; Szmukler-Moncler and coworkers, 2000).

Given a host with normal wound healing, the predictable result for implantation under these conditions should be osseointegration. These factors mirror the concepts proposed by Albrektsson and coworkers (1981).

Previously held recommendations, such as the use of a two-stage procedure, stress-free healing, mucobuccal incisions, sterile conditions, the avoidance of radiographs, and the use of acrylic occlusal surfaces, are no longer considered relevant. Significantly for the discussion of loading protocols, the simple application of force to a healing implant or submucosal healing is only important to the extent that these factors may sometimes lead to excessive implant movement or compromised bacterial control during early healing, interfering with bone growth.

2.2.2   Evolution of Loading Protocols

Several authors and groups have attempted to define loading protocols based on clinical and biological criteria. Conceptually, the groups classified the timing of the introduction of loading during wound healing. The ITI Consensus Conference published its definitions in 2004 (Cochran and coworkers; Chiapasco; Ganeles and Wismeijer; Morton and coworkers), definitions that are similar to those recommended by the Sociedad Española de Implantes World Congress consensus meeting of 2002 in Barcelona, Spain (Aparicio and coworkers, 2003). The ITI group defined loading categories according to the time from the surgical implant placement until the attachment of a prosthetic restoration and according to whether or not the prosthesis was in occlusion. The ITI definitions of the various categories are as follows:

- Conventional loading: A prosthesis attached to the implants in a secondary procedure a minimum of three months following implant placement (it should be noted that when this definition was proposed, it was anticipated that the specific time for healing would be changed over time as implant surfaces and procedures evolved to predictably permit reduced conventional healing times).
- Immediate restoration: A restoration inserted within 48 hours of implant placement, but not in occlusion with the opposing dentition.
- Immediate loading: A restoration placed in occlusion with the opposing dentition within 48 hours of implant placement.
- Early loading: The placement of a restoration in occlusion with the opposing dentition at least 48 hours after implant placement but no later than 3 months afterward.

In a review of clinical studies on early and immediate loading, Attard and Zarb (2005) noted that the long time span incorporated into the definition of early loading (48 hours to 3 months) made this category "tenuous" and that more sensitive and accurate descriptions of healing might be required in the future. Regardless of the concern for the semantics of these loading intervals, they are generally recognized in clinical practice and in the dental literature.

The original loading protocol for osseointegration is currently considered and called conventional loading. There is ample documentation for most dental implant systems to demonstrate that this is a predictable protocol and permits osseointegration (Cochran, 1999; Fugazzotto and coworkers, 2004; Lindh and coworkers, 1998).

A notable exception to this high predictability has been acknowledged with respect to short, machined-surface implants placed in poor-quality bone, particularly in the posterior maxilla. Jaffin and Berman (1991), Hermann and coworkers (2005), and others reported a significantly higher implant loss with shorter, machined-surface implants in the posterior maxilla and mandible. In a broad review of implant surfaces and their effects on healing, Cochran (1999) demonstrated the impact of surface roughness on implant success rates. In the maxilla, rough-surfaced implants had similar success rates in single-tooth and partially dentate applications. He noted that in general, implants in the mandible had a slight advantage in predictability over rough-surfaced implants in the maxilla. Glauser and coworkers (2003) also reported a measurable advantage in success rates when rougher-surfaced implants were used in the maxilla.

Several consensus and review papers have addressed the evolution and predictability of other protocols under different clinical conditions. These reviews include the Barcelona group (Aparicio and coworkers, 2003), the ITI group (Chiapasco, 2004; Ganeles and Wismeijer, 2004; Morton and coworkers, 2004), the European Academy of Osseointegration (Nkenke and Fenner, 2006), the Academy of Osseointegration (Jokstad and Carr, 2007), Gapski and coworkers (2003), Misch and coworkers (2004), Attard and Zarb (2005), Del Fabbro and coworkers (2006), and Ioannidou and coworkers (2005).

When reviewing the literature on loading protocols, it should be recognized that the first significant departures from the conventional approaches were made for edentulous cases. While the focus of this Treatment Guide is on the management of partially dentate patients, there must also be some brief consideration of the evolution and the rationale for the development of loading protocols for edentulous patients.

2.2.3   Edentulous Mandible

Conventional Loading

Conventional loading of implants in the mandible of edentulous patients was the original indication for implant dentistry. Ample data exists to confirm long-term predictability for this treatment modality. Commonly cited references for machined-surface implants include some of the initial publications by Adell and coworkers (1981; 1990). More contemporary implant surfaces and designs also have somewhat better survival/success documentation with expected 5- to 10-year survival rates above 95% (Ferrigno and coworkers, 2002; Behneke and coworkers, 2002; Arvidson and coworkers, 1998; Stoker and coworkers, 2007).

Immediate Loading

English-language reports by several authors about successful immediate loading of fixed restorations included Schnitman and coworkers (1990), Salama and coworkers (1995) and Tarnow and coworkers (1997). These authors generally limited their treatment to fully edentulous mandibles where multiple implants could be placed in dense bone, particularly in the symphyseal region. Immediate fixed restorations were fabricated with reinforced full-arch, one-piece provisionals to rigidly connect the implants and prevent movement during function. Caveats common to most publications include the selection of dense bone for the implant sites, rigid splinting, and the maintenance of the provisionals in the mouth for the duration of healing (Ganeles and coworkers, 2001). Occlusal schemes were created to conform to the principles of "periodontal prosthesis," which were designed to minimize lateral movement of mobile abutment teeth using cross-arch stabilization and rigid splinting (Amsterdam and Abrams, 1973). Adhering to these principles, numerous authors documented hundreds of successful mandibular cases and implants with success rates in the 96% – 100% range, generally equaling those expected of conventional or early loading protocols for edentulous mandibles (Testori and coworkers, 2003; Wolfinger and Balshi, 2003; Horiuchi and coworkers, 2000; Cooper and coworkers, 2002).

Schnitman (1990) reported the highest failure rate of this initial group and noted that the implants that failed were generally short, machined-surface implants located in the posterior mandible, in poor quality bone. Tarnow (1997) noted that the failed implants in his group occurred in conjunction with the periodic removal of the provisional restorations to check implant mobility. When they discontinued removing provisionals as part of their protocol, implant loss ended.

There is ample documentation to support the predictability of immediate loading of four splinted implants for mandibular overdentures, including Babbush (1986) and Chiapasco and coworkers (1997). Additionally, Attard and Zarb (2005) compiled data for mandibular cases constructed with two implants with and without bars indicating high predictability, although they noted that most of the unsplinted implants may not have received full occlusal forces during healing.

Early Loading

Limited documentation is available to evaluate early loading of implants in the fully edentulous mandible, as most publications have addressed either conventional or immediate options. Becker and coworkers (2003) and Ericsson and coworkers (2000) reported high success and survival data comparable to immediate loading protocols. However, in unsplinted overdenture studies, Tawse-Smith and coworkers (2002) indicated some reduction in implant success in early-loaded, machined-surface implants as compared to rough-surface implants. Additional reports of 95% – 100% success rates for rough-surface, unsplinted, early-loaded implants in the mandible are available (Payne and coworkers, 2003; Turkyilmaz and coworkers, 2006).

2.2.4 Edentulous Maxilla

Conventional Loading

Conventional loading of fully edentulous maxillary arches is generally considered predictable, with much documentation available from some of the classic longitudinal implant publications. Lower success rates for implants in the maxilla, as compared to implants in the mandible, have been confirmed with machined-surface implants (Ekfeldt and coworkers, 2001; Jemt and Hager, 2006; Jemt and coworkers, 1996). Jaffin and Berman (1991) and others identified concerns with implants in the maxilla. The use of rough surfaces has been shown to improve maxillary implant survival, but may still show somewhat of a reduction in predictability as compared with mandibular cases (Buser and coworkers, 1997; Ferrigno, 2002). However, some groups reported success rates similar to mandibular cases (Bergkvist and coworkers, 2004). Glauser and coworkers (2003) and Del Fabbro and coworkers (2006) discussed and summarized the improved success rates with rough-surfaced implants in the posterior maxilla.

Immediate Loading

Though far fewer in numbers of cases or implants, several authors reported successful immediate loading of edentulous maxillas (Levine and coworkers, 1998; Jaffin and coworkers, 2004; Ibañez and coworkers, 2005; Gallucci and coworkers, 2004; Ostman and coworkers, 2005). These authors indicate that with proper protocols and patient selection, a high predictability of restorations and cases can be achieved. Recommended techniques for maxillary full-arch immediate loading stress the importance of maximizing implant stability, the use of rough-surfaced, threaded implants, and optimal occlusal control to minimize lateral forces on implants and maximize occlusal stability.

Early Loading

There is a still limited but growing body of information regarding early loading of edentulous maxillary cases. Chiapasco (2004) summarized the limited available data, indicating that early loading of implants in the maxilla in a small series of cases yielded 89% – 100% success rates. Since then, prospective studies by Fischer and coworkers (2004; 2006) and Nordin and coworkers (2004) have indicated very high success and survival rates for implants and fixed restorations with early loading. Jungner and coworkers (2005) compared the effect of roughened-surface implants to that of machined-surface implants under early-loading conditions. Their group noted a small increase in the success rates of roughened implants as compared to machined-surface ones, although the data did not specify success rates for fully edentulous maxillary arches. Raghoebar and coworkers (2003) reported greater than 95% success after 1 year in a group of patients who had bone augmentation followed by overdenture construction, conditions which are thought to reduce the predictability of implants.

2.2.5   Single-Tooth Gaps

Conventional Loading
In Cochran's (1999) meta-analysis of conventionally loaded implants, he confirmed high success rates for rough-surfaced implants placed for single-tooth applications in all areas of the mouth. While the purpose of his review was not to evaluate or compare loading protocols, he was able to summarize data on integration published to that date. Additional reports on the conventional loading of single-tooth implant restorations confirm their high predictability (Levine and coworkers, 1999 and 2002; Haas and coworkers, 2002; Levin and coworkers, 2006a, b). Romeo and coworkers (2002) published a 7-year life-table analysis of 187 single implants. Three implants failed to integrate, while six others were lost during follow-up, resulting in cumulative success and survival rates of, respectively, 93.6% and 96.77%. When only prosthetically loaded implants were considered, the results increased to 96.18% success and 99.35% survival.

Immediate Loading/Restoration
Immediate loading of single-tooth or multi-tooth implant restorations has rarely been reported. Calandriello and coworkers (2003) are among the few authors to intentionally place immediate restorations into direct occlusal contact. They reported 100% survival of all implants at 6 months, with many implants being followed up to 2 years. Instead, the overwhelming majority of documentation for these case types recommends leaving the restorations out of direct occlusal contact during the healing period. Still, the implants are subject to physiologic forces of muscles like the cheek and tongue and to occlusal pressure transmitted through a food bolus.

Numerous authors evaluated success rates and survival rates of immediately restored implants, both in healed ridges and immediately placed in extraction sockets. Table 2 from Ganeles and Wismeijer (2004) summarized much of the data available as of mid-2003. Further publications since 2004 additionally corroborate these data

(Barone and coworkers, 2006; Schwartz-Arad and coworkers, 2007). Of particular note are the few clustered failures reported by some authors, including Ericsson and coworkers (2000), Rocci and coworkers (2003a), and Chaushu and coworkers (2001). The authors concluded that the reduced predictability in sockets was the result of periapical or periodontal pathology present at the time of extraction and implant placement. Yet the implants that were used were either machined-surface or press-fit hydroxylapatite-coated, none of which are currently available.

Early Loading/Restoration
Several studies confirm the high predictability of early loading or restoration of implants in single-tooth sites. These studies were performed with rough-surfaced implants since 2001 by Cochran and coworkers (2002; 2007), Roccuzzo and coworkers (2001), Cooper and coworkers (2001), Testori and coworkers (2002), and others. Most of the reports mixed partially edentulous spans as well as single-tooth replacements. Cooper and coworkers (2001) exclusively focused on anterior single teeth that were restored at approximately 3 weeks, while the others primarily treated posterior sites restored in 6–8 weeks. Turkyilmaz (2006) also reported on maxillary single-tooth replacements and found a success rate of 94% after 3 years. All other authors report success rates of 96%–100% for integration. However, Cochran (2002) and Roccuzzo (2001) noted a few "spinners" that rotated with pain at final abutment connection, but later stabilized after additional healing time. These authors torqued abutment screws to 35 Ncm after 6–8 weeks of healing for type 1, 2, and 3 density bone as part of their protocol. Cooper's group did not note movement of implants, but limited torque to 20 Ncm at 3 weeks.

Roccuzzo and Wilson (2002) reported on a modified surgical protocol for early loading in type 4 posterior maxillary sites. They suggested the use of bone condensation osteotomy preparation followed by unloaded healing. After 6 weeks, a prosthetic abutment was hand-torqued and a provisional restoration was attached out of occlusion. Following an additional 6-week healing period, the abutments were re-torqued to 35 Ncm and a final restoration fabricated and delivered in full occlusion. Using this technique, they achieved approximately 97% implant success.

Common concerns about conventional, immediate, or early loading of single implants principally involve primary implant stability. It is well known for all loading protocols that stability at placement is one of the most significant factors in determining osseointegration or implant failure. When early or immediate loading or restoration is considered for single teeth, this becomes particularly important. There are few opportunities to protect an implant from masticatory or functional forces, leading to deleterious movement before healing is completed. Unlike full-arch restorations, where cross-arch stabilization or multiple unit splinting is possible, single implants must have sufficient primary stability on their own.

Though not readily supportable by dental literature, it can be reasoned that longer, wider implants, with rougher surfaces and larger threads, placed in sites with better bone quality are more likely to have greater stability. Those implants that are placed with less initial stability, whether measured by insertion torque or resonance frequency analysis (RFA), benefit from the longer healing protocols associated with early or conventional loading. No objective studies are available to calculate threshold stability values for each loading protocol. Additionally, it is likely that each manufacturer's implant shapes, surfaces, and designs will exhibit slightly different healing characteristics, making specific loading rules virtually impossible to determine.

Esthetic Factors
More than other clinical applications, single-tooth implant restorations are frequently associated with more stringent esthetic demands. This is probably because if a single tooth is replaced in the maxillary anterior region, there is a presumption that there are usually adjacent natural teeth that must be cosmetically matched. More frequently than with other case types, gingival (pink) esthetics will be relevant for evaluation of success. Volume I of the ITI Treatment Guide discusses esthetic considerations for implant dentistry in depth (Buser and coworkers, 2006).

The requirements for this restoration type become more stringent than merely achieving physiologic homeostasis with soft and hard tissue. Additionally, the factors associated with implant esthetics become relevant (Buser and coworkers, 2004; Belser and coworkers, 2004; Grunder and coworkers, 2005). Logically, it can be proposed that in sites where teeth are extracted without significant alveolar damage, earlier restoration protocols would seem to be able to preserve gingival architecture better than conventional ones. In more conventional or delayed protocols, gingival contours and papillary forms need to be reestablished through grafting and contouring procedures. Several authors documented esthetic changes following immediate implant placement and restoration, generally finding short-term recession of 0.5–1 mm (Kan and coworkers, 2003; Hui and coworkers, 2001), which was not deemed to be of great significance. More importantly, these observations of tissue changes are consistent with recession measurements taken of implants allowed to heal with conventional loading protocols (Grunder, 2002; Small and Tarnow, 2000; Choquet and coworkers, 2001; Priest, 2003; Juodzbalys and Wang, 2007), indicating that

early or immediate restoration by itself may not affect the esthetic results of treatment.

While there is ample evidence to anticipate that single implants immediately restored in the esthetic zone will achieve integration, there is considerably less data to rely on to predict positive esthetic results. A careful esthetic risk assessment (Buser and coworkers, 2006) must be combined with site analysis to determine the most appropriate loading protocol. If an accelerated protocol is considered, the importance and predictability of any augmentation procedure should be assessed and considered in determining an appropriate restoration or loading time.

2.2.6 Multi-Tooth Gaps

Conventional Loading
Much of the literature that addresses partial edentulism often does not differentiate between the replacement of single teeth or multiple teeth in a short span. Biomechanically, the conditions are similar for both situations if the teeth to be replaced are in the same quadrant. These implants and restorations cannot gain support from cross-arch stabilization or the direction of lateral forces around the line of an arc, as full-arch restorations might. Instead, they rely predominantly on primary stability from the implant interactions with the surrounding osteotomy, until secondary healing occurs.

There is ample data to confirm the efficacy of conventional loading in partially dentate cases. Lindh and coworkers (1998) published a meta-analysis of partially dentate cases, indicating a success rate of 85.7% for implants and a survival rate of 93.6% after 6–7 years. Lekholm and coworkers (1999) reported a 10-year survival rate of 92.6% on machined-surfaced implants placed between July 1985 and April 1987. The cumulative survival rate of implants was 90.2% in the maxilla and 92.6% in the mandible. Naert and coworkers (2002) reported a 91.4% cumulative survival rate on 1956 machined-surface implants that were used in partially dentate patients and followed up to 16 years. Other authors report improved success and/or survival data with newer implant systems over shorter time intervals. These include Buser and coworkers (1997), Fugazzotto and coworkers (2004), and others, who have shown up to 99% survival for up to 7 years.

Immediate Restoration/Loading
Similar to the management of single teeth, multi-unit restorations are typically not placed into full occlusal function. Almost all available literature relates to immediate restoration rather than immediate loading. An exception to this trend is a recent publication by Schincaglia and

coworkers (2007), who placed restorations into "light centric occlusal contact." Their study was a randomized, controlled trial, in which patients received immediately loaded, implant-supported posterior mandibular fixed dental prosthesis. One side received machined-surface implants while the other received oxidized-surface implants. They also recorded the maximum insertion torque and implant stability quotient (ISQ) values. After 1 year of function, 20/22 machined-surface implants were successful while 20/20 oxidized-surface implants were successful. ISQ and insertion torque values for both groups of implants were similar. The authors concluded that oxidized-surface implants placed in the posterior mandible, inserted with ≥20 Ncm and ISQ value ≥60 can be immediately loaded in partially dentate patients in many circumstances.

Rocci and coworkers (2003b) also documented an increased success rate with oxidized-surface implants as compared to machined-surface ones in partially dentate cases. There are other reports of immediately restored implants in partially dentate patients. Many authors have reported high success rates, including Calandriello and coworkers (2003) and Degidi and Piattelli (2003). Among their recommendations is to plan cases with a large number of implants. Calandriello recommended one implant per tooth, while Degidi recommended a ratio of 1.4 or 1.5 teeth per implant in the maxilla and mandible respectively. These formulae were not evidence-based, but rather represented the clinical judgment of the authors. None of the studies on partially dentate cases focused on esthetic results and none addressed the use of reduced diameter implants, which may be indicated in the mandibular incisor area.

Early Loading
Several authors have documented high predictability with the early restoration protocols. Roccuzzo and coworkers (2001) prospectively evaluated TPS-surfaced implants loaded conventionally with sandblasted, acid-etched implants at 6 weeks. The results were that 4 of 68 early-loading Straumann SLA implants did not withstand full torque application at 6 weeks, but then proceeded to heal uneventfully after another 6 weeks. At 1 year, all implants were successfully in function. Cochran and coworkers (2002), Testori and coworkers (2002), and Nordin and coworkers (2004) also reported on early loading of microtextured-surface implants showing survival rates exceeding 97%. In a multi-center clinical trial, Cochran and coworkers (2007) reported implant survival of >99% at 3 and 5 years for sandblasted, acid-etched implants restored in an early loading protocol. It should be noted that an exclusion criterion for the above studies was poor bone quality, which delayed the loading until 3 months after placement, which is considered conventional loading.

Jungner and coworkers (2005) studied the results of patients treated with different implant surfaces and loading protocols. He found 100% integration for the oxidized-surface implants with early or conventional loading, but 7 of 195 machined-surface implants failed. No statistical analysis was performed, but the trend was favorable towards the roughened surface, despite the more aggressive loading protocol. Similar results were reported by Gotfredsen and Karlsson (2001), who placed fixed dental prosthesis so that each restoration was supported by at least one early-loaded machined and one grit-blasted implant. They found after 5 years that 3 of 64 (4.9%) machined-surface implants failed, but none of the roughened-surface implants failed. All other clinical parameters between the groups were similar.

2.2.7   Conclusion

From reviewing the scientific literature, it is clear that there is an abundance of case reports and case series relating to implant success or survival and loading protocols. Some well-planned and well-conducted studies with the statistical power to draw factual conclusions are beginning to appear in this field. Yet, the majority of the information cannot be scientifically analyzed. Recent attempts to draw conclusions about implant success and loading protocols by Jokstad and Carr (2007), Del Fabbro and coworkers (2006), Attard and Zarb (2005), Nkenke and Fenner (2006), and Ioannidou and Doufexi (2006) yielded few solid conclusions.

Certainly, strong inferences can be drawn from the body of information. These include:

- Implants can heal under loaded and unloaded conditions, provided that certain factors are controlled in all case types.
- There appears to be an adequate body of knowledge to suggest that immediate loading of a fully edentulous mandible is a reasonable treatment option, provided other patient factors are positive.
- Roughened-surface implants appear to have higher success rates than machined-surface implants under all loading conditions.
- Immobilizing implants through primary stability during healing is critical to successful osseointegration.
- An adequate number and distribution of implants is needed for successful outcomes.
- Immediate placement of implants, with or without provisional restorations, may lead to buccal bone loss and gingival recession, which could be esthetically significant in some patients.

Information that is not readily apparent from the literature includes:

- The authors of the articles are among the most skilled and experienced surgeons and restorative dentists in the field, with optimal resources for complex treatments.
- Their results for riskier procedures, such as immediate loading, may not be easily duplicated by less experienced or knowledgeable clinicians.
- The reported results are from patients pre-selected for successful outcomes. Skilled, experienced clinicians perform their own risk assessment, excluding inappropriate patients. Currently, there are no published risk assessment guidelines to assist in determining loading protocols.
- Some case types are more easily accomplished than others, even though success rates may be similar. For example, immediately loaded complete mandibular cases are easier to treat than immediately loaded full maxillary cases.
- Threshold values for primary stability for immediate or early loading, as measured by ISQ or insertion torque for osseointegration, are unknown.
- The optimal number, distribution, and location of implants, given specific case types, has not yet been described.

- The influence of systemic conditions or illness such as age, diabetes, steroid use, osteoporosis, or metabolic disorder has not been considered as they relate to loading protocols.
- The influence of different loading protocols on grafted bone is unknown.
- The influence of environmental factors, such as smoking or bruxism, with respect to loading protocol is not well reported.
- The influence of biotype on osseointegration and tissue stability as related to loading protocol is unknown.
- The influence of periodontal status and the implications of immediate placement on long-term success loading is unknown.

Ultimately, it is the responsibility of each clinician to create an algorithm for him- or herself to help in providing treatment. This formula should combine the patient's diagnosis and expectations with the clinician's experience, ability, and knowledge, plus available resources to provide therapeutic solutions. Familiarity with the scientific literature is an essential component of this equation.

3 General Principles for the Pre-Treatment Assessment of and Planning for Partially Dentate Patients Receiving Dental Implants

D. Morton, W. C. Martin, D. Buser

3.1 Summary of Treatment Risk Profile

Treatment planning for partially dentate patients is critical to achieving optimum outcomes considered satisfactory by both patients and clinicians. Many factors should routinely be considered during the planning process in an effort to improve the predictability of treatment. Treatment regulators are the major factors that influence the presence or absence of risk to successful treatment outcomes. Each regulator is characterized by factors capable of reducing the quality of the treatment, and as such should be objectively evaluated for each treatment indication.

The following table summarizes the risk factors associated with the treatment of partially dentate patients (Table 1). Based on a detailed preoperative analysis, the individual risk profile of each patient can be established.

Table 1   Risk Factors Associated with the Treatment of Partially Dentate Patients.

Treatment Regulator	Risk Factor	Degree of Risk		
		Low	Medium	High
Clinician	Skill and education	Experienced clinician with formal postgraduate training or high levels of implant-specific continuing education	Experienced clinician with moderate levels of implant-specific continuing education	Inexperienced clinician with limited implant-specific continuing education
	Experience	Extensive implant-specific clinical experience	Moderate implant-specific clinical experience	Limited implant-specific clinical experience
Patient	Medical risk factors	Absence of medical risk factors	Medical conditions present though controlled	Medical conditions that retard or diminish implant integration and smoking
	Dental risk factors	Absence of periodontal or occlusal disease, high levels of hygiene and compliance	History of controlled periodontal or occlusal disease, questionable oral hygiene or compliance	Active periodontal or occlusal disease, poor levels of hygiene and compliance
	Anatomic risk factors	Type 1 and 2 bone, adequate interocclusal space, favorable opposing dentition	Type 3 bone, questionable interocclusal space, less than ideal opposing dentition	Type 4 bone, inadequate interocclusal space, unfavorable malocclusion
	Esthetic risk factors	Low esthetic risk based on esthetic risk profile	Moderate esthetic risk profile based on esthetic risk profile	High esthetic risk based on esthetic risk profile
Surgical approach	Documentation and evidence	Type 3 and 4 implant placement when implants with a micro-roughened surface are used	Type 2 implant placement when implants with a micro-roughened surface are used	Type 1 (immediate) placement when implants with a micro-roughened surface are used
Difficulty	SAC classification	Straightforward	Advanced	Complex

3.2   Treatment Regulators and Risk Factors

The most critical regulator capable of determining the quality of the treatment is the clinician. The clinician's skill, ability to pay meticulous attention to detail, and experience must not be underestimated. Clinicians with advanced training in oral surgery, periodontology and/or prosthodontics or with high levels of implant-specific continuing education are often better prepared to provide treatment for patients whose treatment presents medium or high risk.

Clinicians with moderate levels of clinical experience and continuing education in implant and comprehensive dentistry should be encouraged to manage the rehabilitation of patients with low and medium risk to outcomes. These clinicians are more likely to recognize the need for specialty involvement and will most likely embrace accepted protocols, including a team approach to treatment and restoration-based implant treatment philosophies.

Inexperienced clinicians with only limited exposure to implant-specific continuing education should limit treatments to low-risk patients. These clinicians should seek access to experienced mentors and further education if they desire to increase levels of treatment difficulty.

A team approach to patient planning and treatment should be encouraged where at all possible in order to improve the opportunity for clinicians to gather experience and education with no concurrent risk to patients and their treatment success.

Another critical treatment regulator is the patient. The medical status of the patient should always be evaluated as part of the pre-treatment analysis. Because the loading of dental implants transfers stress to the supporting structures, particular emphasis should be placed on systemic disorders capable of reducing this capacity. Such factors may include diabetes, immune diseases, bone diseases, and smoking.

The dental status of the patient is a primary concern. The presence or absence of periodontal disease (both past and present) and the patient's response to therapy should be noted. The patient's occlusal classification and the presence or absence of occlusal disease is also important. The capacity to distribute occlusal loads appropriately through the stomatognathic system with the planned definitive restoration or restorations should be routinely evaluated.

The patients' level of hygiene and motivation towards their dental health also influences treatment risk. Those patients with less than ideal oral hygiene and low motivation should have behavioral modification prior to the commencement of implant-based care. This risk factor is important to the health and integrity of the entire dentition, not only to the planned implants and restorations.

Lastly, the local anatomy of the site is an important consideration when evaluating the restorative phase of treatment. Patients characterized by type 1 and 2 bone, where high levels of implant survival are routinely observed, can be treated with a variety of loading options at a relatively low risk (Table 2). Risk to implant survival, particularly in the early stages of healing, increases as the quality of the supporting bone diminishes. Most implant failures continue to be recorded prior to, or shortly after, restorative loading, and are often associated with reduced bone

Table 2   Lekholm and Zarb Classification of Bone Density/Quality (Lekholm and Zarb, 1985).

Compact Bone	Trabecular Bone	Type (Bone Density/Quality)
Homogenous compact bone throughout the entire jaw	Small amount of dense trabecular bone	1
Thick layer of compact bone	Core of dense trabecular bone	2
Thin rim of cortical bone	Core of dense trabecular bone	3
Thin rim of cortical bone	Core of low-density trabecular bone	4

quality or regions characterized by such. Emphasis should be placed on the combination of implant surface area and bone quality, as short implants in type 3 and 4 bone can result in higher treatment risk for some implant systems, particularly when combined with accelerated treatment protocols (Table 2). More mature bone may be recommended in such circumstances.

Partially dentate patients can also have their planned treatment classified as straightforward, advanced, or complex. This classification, first presented by the Swiss Society for Implantology and the subject of a recent ITI Consensus Conference, objectively recognizes the oral condition of the patient and the likely difficulty of treatment.

Traditionally, implants have only been loaded if the tissues were considered healthy and if adequate stability could be confirmed. Unfortunately, apparent implant health and immobility have become synonymous with the term 'osseointegration'. This is, however, inaccurate, as the original definition of osseointegration required the implant to support functional load. Implants can be capable of supporting load immediately upon placement if they are stable and if the prevailing conditions are otherwise favorable. The same can be said for early restoration and loading, particularly if the implants are characterized by modern roughened or chemically modified implant surfaces. It should be noted that implants placed immediately into extraction sites, or into immature healing sites, ultimately survive. Evidence of their long-term capacity to support a restoration deemed satisfactory to the patient and clinician is less compelling. It is for this reason that recommendations made in this guide assume healthy and stable implants at the time of loading. The influence of placement chronology on treatment outcome will be considered in a later volume.

Conventional and early loading of implants placed in regions of single missing teeth in posterior sites are considered straightforward for several reasons (Fig 1). Firstly, the

patient's desires are often limited to improved masticatory function and the prevention of food impaction in the implant space. The simple provision of a restoration will satisfy most of these patients. In addition, their demands in terms of esthetics, phonetics, facial support, and self-esteem are low. The adjacent teeth and the remaining dentition often provide additional support for the occlusion, lessening the likelihood of occlusal overload.

Restorative procedures familiar to the clinician are also indicated for such restorations. Cemented restorations, with minimally demanding component selection, can be utilized with low risk. Provisional restorations, while recommended in most circumstances, are not critical to the outcome. Minor variations in implant position are readily addressed with no critical compromise to restorative capability.

The immediate restoration of single implants in posterior regions is considered advanced. Additional care and attention to detail is required because the healing of the bone and surrounding soft tissues can be influenced by the quality of the restoration and the management of load. Occlusal harmony is of particular importance, as the initial stability of the implant will diminish throughout the early weeks of healing. Occlusal load is capable of inducing undesirable movement of the implant during this period, with the possibility of implant failure. Management of load distribution through occlusal design and treatment technique requires higher levels of skill and experience from the clinician.

The restoration of single missing teeth in the anterior region of the mouth is more complicated and falls into the advanced or complex categories, depending on the loading protocol (Fig 2). The need for an esthetic outcome is paramount for many patients and appropriate preoperative analysis requires an assessment of esthetic risk, as detailed in Volume 1 of the ITI Treatment Guide. Simple survival of the implant and restoration is inadequate and does not guarantee a favorable outcome. Restorations

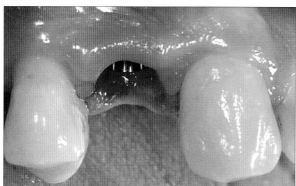

Fig 1   Single-tooth replacement of tooth 14 with a dental implant.

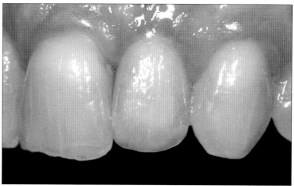

Fig 2   Four-year follow-up of an implant restoration of tooth 22.

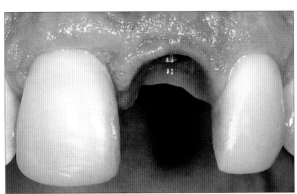

Fig 3   Developed transition zone around site 21.

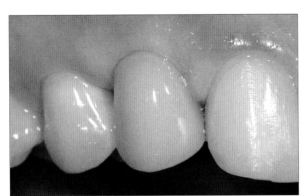

Fig 4   Immediate restoration of an implant in site 13.

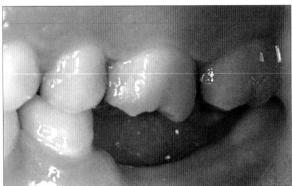

Fig 5   Limited interocclusal space for implant placement and restoration at site 36–37.

must be in harmony with the face and smile of the patient, must be associated with a healthy surrounding periodontium (both in the short and long term), and must accurately mimic the lost tooth with regard to color, optical properties, and form (Belser and coworkers, 2004). Achieving these goals requires clinicians to have a greater depth of knowledge, not only in implant dentistry but in esthetic dentistry as well.

Of particular importance is a clear understanding of the soft tissues and their behavior. The response of the transition zone (from the restorative margin of the implant to the mucosal margin in the oral cavity) to the restoration is often the factor limiting or providing treatment success (Fig 3).

Restoring implants in the esthetic zone demands a more detailed knowledge of components and their use. Since the gingival architecture is more scalloped in shape, the use of machined and screw-retained components at the level of the implant is indicated for both provisional and definitive restorations. This can often complicate prosthesis design, impression-making, and laboratory procedures.

The immediate restoration of single implants in the anterior regions, particularly of the maxilla, is considered complex (Fig 4). The highest level of knowledge with regard to soft tissue response is required. Overcontoured and undercontoured provisional restorations can lead to irreversible changes in soft tissue form, in turn resulting in esthetic compromise. While an excellent soft-tissue response can be achieved with immediate provisional restorations, such procedures should be undertaken only by the most experienced, skilled, and educated clinicians because of the esthetic risk associated with them.

The replacement of adjacent missing teeth with implant-supported restorations is more challenging. In the posterior regions of the mouth, additional challenges are often associated with impression procedures and technical difficulty. Treatment planning of individual implant-supported restorations, or implant-supported fixed dental prostheses, requires a higher degree of knowledge. The opposing dentition, interocclusal space, and implant position each increase the treatment difficulty (Fig 5). The prevailing occlusal scheme is also important as anterior guidance can in some cases assist the clinician in controlling occlusal load, whereas group function (particularly in bruxing patients) can be difficult to manage.

The immediate restoration of adjacent implants in the posterior regions of the mouth is considered complex. These restorations are often required to bear a greater functional load and are less protected by the remaining dentition. In addition, the need for the appropriate passivity of the provisional restoration adds to the skills required of the clinician and, where involved, of the technician. The patient benefit of such procedures should be identified prior to treatment, with particular emphasis placed on the possible loss of the implants.

In the anterior regions of the mouth, particularly where the esthetic outcome is critical, treatment is far more complicated. For clinicians with high levels of implant and esthetic training, conventional and early loading can be considered advanced. A restoration-driven, three-dimensional approach to implant placement is a pre-requisite for treatment in this area, as the position of the implant and the surgical method employed may be the single most influential factor affecting the restorative outcome.

The provisional restoration of implants placed in regions of adjacent missing teeth in the anterior regions of the mouth is mandatory in order to ensure the maturation of the transition zone and the development of the optimal emergence profile and tissue form. The degree of technical difficulty for these patients is increased by the need for screw retention in most circumstances, and the need for accurate impression-making and technical procedures.

The immediate restoration of implants placed in areas of adjacent missing teeth in the anterior maxilla should be reserved for the most experienced implant clinicians, who have the requisite knowledge of esthetic dental principles. While it remains clear that the benefits of immediate provisional restoration or loading may be considerable to the patient, the risk of permanent soft tissue loss cannot be overemphasized. Further, the immediate restoration of implants in the anterior regions of the mouth may be associated with unreasonable risk to implant survival, as control of off-axis load is more difficult. Therefore, patient compliance is a major factor to be considered in pre-treatment assessment.

The surgical approach to implant placement, while not a primary consideration of this treatment guide, cannot be excluded as a factor to be considered in the pre-treatment assessment of these patients. Immediate (type 1) implant placement has been associated with predictable survival, but the response of the soft tissues and facial supporting bone remain controversial (Hämmerle and coworkers, 2004). The restoration of implants associated with immature supporting hard and soft tissues can be complicated by the response to the surgery in addition to the factors mentioned above. Conventional and early loading is therefore recommended for the majority of patients who have received immediate implant placement, so that the tissue response to implant placement can be observed. Only in the rarest of circumstances should the immediate restoration or loading of immediately placed implants be considered, and it is recommended only for clinicians with the highest levels of education, judgment, and skill.

The implant and restorative components chosen to support the restoration are critical to the decision-making process. Conventional restoration and loading protocols were associated with machined implants, and were largely designed to comply with time-related implant survival rates. As implant surfaces and connections have evolved, loading protocols have also been modified. Many of the changes to loading recommendations have been supported by basic, animal, and clinical research prior to their routine clinical application. Microroughened implant surfaces are well-documented with regard to loading and restoration times of 6–8 weeks (early). Where possible, clinicians considering immediate or early loading of implants should utilize this scientific evidence with regard to implant selection. Further enhancement of the implant surface seems promising. Chemically modified implant surfaces are proving capable of supporting occlusal load with immediate and early loading protocols, though data is to date small in number and short in term. The influence of the implant surface, though, is increasing as it relates to loading protocols.

3.3 Factors Influencing Decision-Making in Treatment Approaches

Dental implants can be loaded at varying time intervals subsequent to placement. The decision to utilize immediate, early, or conventional loading protocols should be based on careful evaluation of the patient, as noted above, and on each individual situation. This chapter is intended to identify and discuss important factors that may influence the clinician's choice for an appropriate treatment approach with regard to loading in a given clinical circumstance.

These factors can be divided into five categories:

- The body (quantity and quality) of scientific documentation supporting the treatment approach.
- The benefit to the patient associated with the treatment approach.
- The risk for complication associated with the treatment approach.
- The treatment difficulty associated with the treatment approach.
- The cost-effectiveness of the treatment approach.

Patient treatments will be provided in Chapter 4 of this volume of the ITI Treatment Guide. Treatments will be classified according to site (maxillary and mandibular distal extensions, anterior and posterior single missing teeth, and anterior extended edentulous regions), and loading protocol (conventional, early, or immediate). The factors noted above will be used to allow the comparison of loading options for each clinical indication, and to facilitate the development of meaningful recommendations for loading in each clinical indication.

3.3.1   Scientific Documentation

All clinical procedures associated with implant-based treatment should be well-supported by scientific evidence. While it is understood that there are different levels of evidence, this treatment guide will use a simplified interpretation of the available evidence and will consider in conjunction the time and degree of the documentation. The goal is to allow for the development of useful and clinically applicable conclusions and recommendations.

A loading protocol is considered well-documented when clinical studies with a follow-up of at least five years have been published in peer-reviewed journals. A procedure is considered moderately documented when only short to medium-range clinical studies (1 – 3 years) are available.

Procedures are scientifically not documented when no clinical studies, or only case reports, have been published.

3.3.2   Benefit for the Patient

It is appropriate that all clinical decisions are based on providing a benefit for the patient. Reduced treatment time through early or immediate loading protocols can be considered beneficial to the patient. Patient comfort and masticatory function during the healing period can be improved with early or immediate placement of implant-supported provisional restorations. This benefit is maximized by immediate loading protocols in appropriate clinical indications.

Esthetic advantages may also be observed with early or immediate loading protocols, particularly in the anterior maxilla. This advantage has been associated with enhanced soft tissue conditioning, shaping, and maturation to optimize esthetic outcomes when compared to conventional loading protocols. The benefit to the patient associated with loading options and site will be categorized as high, moderate, or low in the patient presentations in Chapter 4.

It is important to note that early and immediate loading protocols can be associated with an increased incidence and/or severity of complications, including bone and soft tissue loss and the consequent lack of esthetic predictability. On rare occasions, accelerated loading protocols have been associated with early implant loss. Any benefits need to be carefully considered with regard to possible complications.

3.3.3   Risk for Complications

Immediate and early loading protocols can be associated with an increased risk of treatment complications. The most important complication of immediate and early loading is early implant failure. This can often be explained by overload of the bone-to-implant interface during the healing phase, leading to excessive micromotion. The quantity and quality of bone, and the capacity to maintain implant stability, is an important consideration. These factors often vary in different regions of the mouth or when augmentation procedures have been utilized; this should be considered when selecting a loading option. In addition, a differentiation between splinted and non-splinted implants (effective distribution of load) should be made.

In the anterior regions of the maxilla, esthetic complications are primary concerns. Such complications can be the result of less than ideal hard and soft tissue healing. The predictability of the tissue response to immediate and early loading can be questionable. A comprehensive esthetic risk assessment, with particular reference to tissue biotype and hard and soft tissue deficits, should be undertaken when considering a particular loading protocol in this region.

The risk for complications associated with loading protocols can be increased by additional factors. General and dental health conditions, in addition to the anatomic and surgical aspects of treatment, can increase these risks. Health factors of significance include systemic and oral diseases. The timing of implant placement with regard to extraction, and the presence or absence of hard and/or soft tissue grafting procedures, will influence the available loading options and the level of risk associated with them.

3.3.4 Difficulty Level of the Prosthodontic Treatment

The restorative or prosthodontic phase of therapy can be divided into straightforward, advanced, and complex categories, depending on the objective pre-treatment assessment of the patient. Factors of significance can be both general and restoration-specific. General factors include the medical health status of the patient, their psychosocial circumstances, and whether they smoke or not.

Factors specific to the restorative treatment include skeletal jaw relationships, symmetry in the anterior maxilla, the space available for restorative materials, mesiodistal and orofacial dimensions of the edentulous region, the periodontal, occlusal and parafunctional status of the patient, the position of the implant or implants, and the esthetic risk.

3.3.5 Cost-Effectiveness

The overall cost of treatment is a great concern for most patients. The cost is influenced by the preoperative planning, the surgical and prosthetic procedures, implant components and biomaterials as well as laboratory expenses. Straightforward procedures tend to be less expensive, while more advanced and complex procedures involving multiple treatment steps normally increase the cost. Therefore, where possible, patients should be provided with cost-effective treatment options that optimize outcomes and control the risk of complications.

4 <u>Clinical Case Presentations Based on Different Loading Protocols</u>

Posterior Multi-Tooth Gaps and Free-End Situations in the Maxilla or Mandible

4.1 Replacement of Multiple Teeth in a Partially Dentate Posterior Mandible with a Fixed Dental Prosthesis Using an Early Loading Protocol

Y. Nakajima

A 55-year-old female patient was referred for consultation and treatment. Her chief complaint was pain associated with the mandibular right second premolar (tooth 45). The patient denied systemic or oral diseases capable of compromising dental care. She had a history of adult periodontitis, for which she continued to be treated. Her response to therapy and motivation towards dental health were considered excellent.

Intraoral examination revealed a cantilever fixed dental prosthesis in the mandibular right quadrant, with retainers on teeth 45 and 47, and pontics at sites 44 and 46. The retainer on tooth 45 was loose, and the tooth was carious. Radiographic evaluation confirmed the extent of the caries and the maintenance of bone around tooth 45 and in the pontic region 46 (Fig 1).

Removal of the fixed dental prosthesis revealed the extent of the destruction of tooth 45, which was considered to be non-restorable (Fig 2).

The patient was given several treatment options. These included:

- Option 1: Bone augmentation at site 44, to be followed by implant placement in sites 44, 45, and 46. This would allow for single-tooth implant-supported crowns in sites 44, 45, and 46, and a metal-ceramic crown on tooth 47.

- Option 2: Bone augmentation at site 44, to be followed by implant placement in sites 44 and 46. This would facilitate restoration with an implant-supported fixed dental prosthesis (44 – 46), and a metal ceramic crown on tooth 47.

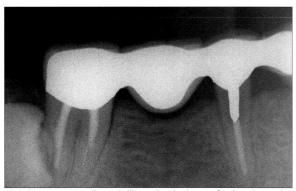

Fig 1 Pretreatment radiograph, illustrating the degree of carious destruction involvment on tooth 45 and the bone height around tooth 45 and under the pontic at site 46.

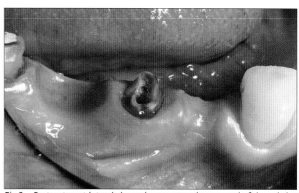

Fig 2 Pretreatment lateral view subsequent to the removal of the existing fixed dental prosthesis.

- Option 3: Placement of dental implants in sites 45 and 46. This would allow for the fabrication of a fixed dental prosthesis (44 – 46) with a cantilevered unit (44). A metal-ceramic crown would be provided on tooth 47.

- Option 4: The fabrication of a conventional removable partial denture.

The patient chose not to augment site 44, and she preferred a fixed restoration. After considering all the treatment options, the patient elected and consented to pursue treatment option 3 (two implants and a cantilevered fixed dental prosthesis). Immediate (type 1) implant placement in site 45 was to be undertaken, should hard and soft tissue volume be considered adequate after the extraction of the tooth.

Tooth 45 was extracted with periotomes and elevators without incident. Trauma to surrounding soft tissues and bone was minimized and the site was considered appropriate for the immediate placement of a dental implant. A full thickness mucoperiosteal flap was elevated, and two Straumann Standard Plus implants were positioned in sites 45 (endosteal diameter, 4.1 mm; length, 10 mm; Regular Neck prosthetic platform, 4.8 mm) and 46 (endosteal diameter, 4.8 mm; length, 10 mm; Wide Neck prosthetic platform, 6.5 mm) according to a restoration-driven protocol, using appropriate templates. Both implants were considered stable, and the dimension of the horizontal defect surrounding the implant in site 45 was less than 1 mm (Fig 3).

Healing caps were then positioned to ensure transmucosal healing, and the wound was sutured closed (Fig 4).

After 6 weeks of healing, the patient was evaluated and the soft tissue response was considered excellent (Fig 5).

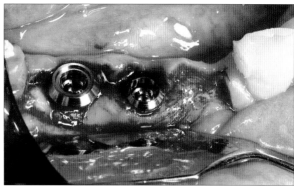

Fig 3   After implant placement. Note the restorative margins at the height of the buccal bone crests and the limited horizontal defect.

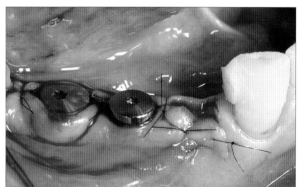

Fig 4   The implants with the healing caps and wound closure.

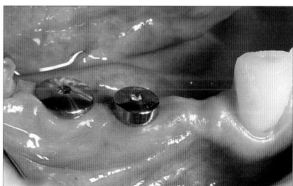

Fig 5   The healing caps and soft tissue healing 6 weeks after implant placement.

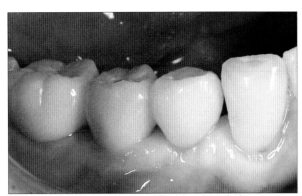

Fig 6   The screw-retained provisional fixed dental prosthesis.

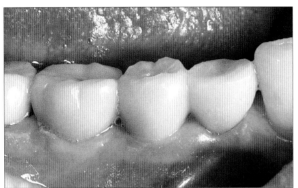

Fig 7   The screw-retained provisional fixed dental prosthesis 6 weeks after placement.

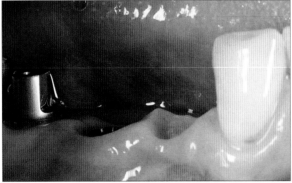

Fig 8   Soft-tissue condition after 6 weeks of provisional restoration.

The healing caps were removed, and the sulcus depth on both implants was considered to be less than 3 mm in all areas. Impression caps were positioned to allow for the registration of the implant shoulders, and appropriate positioning cylinders were then placed without incident. A polyvinyl siloxane impression was made to facilitate the indirect fabrication of the provisional restoration. The screw-retained provisional restoration was fabricated in acrylic resin incorporating titanium provisional cylinders for bridges, and it was delivered 8 weeks after implant placement without incident (Fig 6). The cantilevered unit was kept out of occlusion in centric relation and all excursions. Transient blanching (less than 10 minutes) was observed in the region of the ovate pontic.

The soft tissues adjacent to the provisional restoration were allowed to mature for an additional 6 weeks (Fig 7). The health of all tissues was confirmed subsequent to removal of the provisional restoration (Fig 8).

A customized impression cap, duplicating the emergence of the restoration at site 45, and the ovate site 44, was then fabricated (Fig 9) and positioned (Fig 10). A final impression was then taken in polyvinyl siloxane and a cast poured.

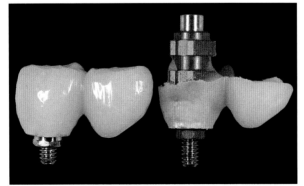

Fig 9   The customized screw-retained synOcta impression cap and duplicated ovate pontic.

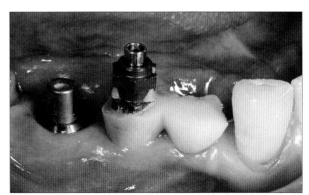

Fig 10   The customized impression cap in position.

A high-strength, biocompatible cementable zirconium oxide framework (Zeno-Tec) was fabricated on the customized master cast, utilizing 2-piece cementable synOcta abutments (Fig 11). Attention to tooth position, room for veneering ceramic, and connector dimension was required to provide adequate resistance to fracture, particularly in the cantilever region. Feldspathic ceramic was then applied to the framework (Fig 12). The emergence profile of the restoration was carefully controlled to prevent inappropriate contouring and to improve the esthetic outcome (Fig 13).

At delivery, the occlusal, esthetic, and hygienic results were confirmed and modified as required (Fig 14). The cementable synOcta abutments were torqued to 35 Ncm without incident and the final prosthesis permanently luted using glass- ionomer cement (Fig 15). The patient was placed on a 3-month recall schedule and was completely satisfied with the outcome.

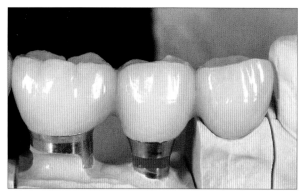

Fig 12   The final fixed dental prosthesis on the master cast.

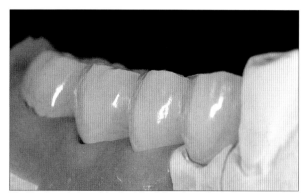

Fig 13   Buccal view of the final fixed dental prosthesis, illustrating an appropriate emergence profile.

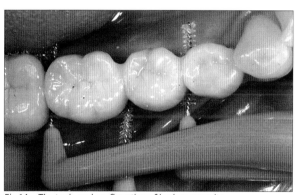

Fig 14   The try-in and confirmation of hygiene capacity.

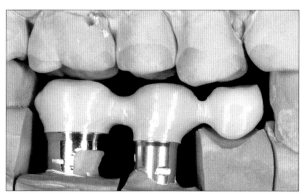

Fig 11   High-strength biocompatible zirconium oxide framework, illustrating adequate room for feldspathic ceramic and connector dimensions.

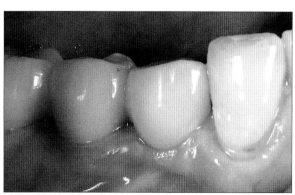

Fig 15   The fixed dental prosthesis immediately subsequent to cementation.

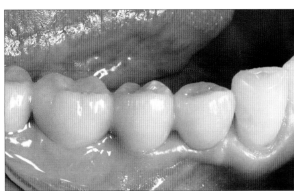

Fig 16   The fixed dental prosthesis at the 18-month follow-up appointment.

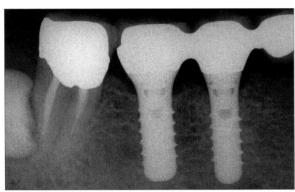

Fig 17   Periapical radiograph 18 months after placement of the prosthesis. Bone levels adjacent to the implants and in the ovate pontic region appear excellent.

At the 18-month recall visit, oral hygiene maintenance was considered excellent and the fixed dental prosthesis was free of complications (Fig 16).

The periapical radiograph 18 months after implant restoration confirmed excellent bone maintenance (Fig 17).

Acknowledgments

Laboratory Procedures
Isamu Saitou – CDT, IS Dental, Tokyo, Japan.

Oral Hygienist
Yuki Seki – DH, Nakajima Dental Clinic.

4.2 Replacement of Multiple Teeth in a Partially Dentate Posterior Mandible with a Fixed Dental Prosthesis Using an Early Loading Protocol

W. C. Martin, J. Ruskin

In 2002, a 27-year-old female patient was referred to our clinic for the treatment of her failing dentition. The patient's medical history revealed no significant findings that would preclude routine dental procedures. She reported no drug allergies and was currently taking no medications. Her dental history was restricted to operative dentistry that addressed several areas of recurrent decay. The patient was on a periodontal recall and home care program that continually fell short of maintaining a healthy dentition. The patient's chief complaint was: "My teeth often break, and they are sensitive when I eat and drink."

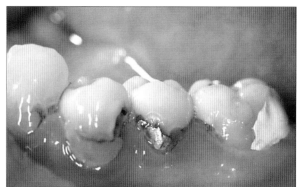

Fig 1   Lateral view of teeth 33 – 36.

An intraoral examination revealed several areas of recurrent decay around restorations that were placed within a 3-year period. The majority of the teeth in quadrants 1 to 3 were restorable without the need for endodontic or periodontal intervention. Teeth 33 – 36 exhibited gross recurrent decay with severe gingival inflammation (Fig 1). Tooth 36 had circumferential decay extending from the distolingual surface to the distofacial, with occlusal involvement. In addition, the decay extended approximately 3 mm subgingivally. Tooth 35 exhibited facial and subgingival recurrent decay with occlusal caries. Tooth 34 exhibited facial recurrent decay extending 2 mm subgingivally with occlusal caries. Tooth 33 exhibited facial recurrent decay extending 1 mm subgingivally.

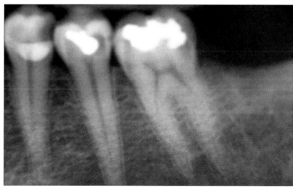

Fig 2   Periapical radiograph of teeth 34 – 36.

The radiographic analysis of teeth 34 – 36 confirmed the findings of recurrent decay (Fig 2). There were no radiographic signs of bone loss or of the widening of the periodontal ligament space. The pulp chambers and canals were visible and there were no signs of periapical radiolucencies. The teeth tested vital to an electric pulp test.

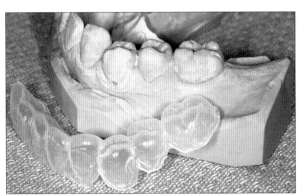

Fig 3a   A vacuform template (6 mm) of the existing teeth was fabricated.

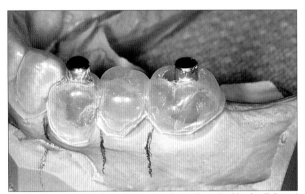

Fig 3b   The cast was adjusted to remove the teeth, and guide pins (3.5 mm) were placed in ideal restorative positions based upon the planned restoration and existing ridge shape.

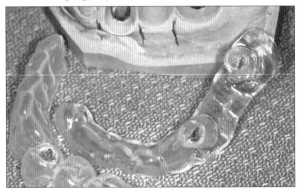

Fig 3c   A vacuform template (2 mm) was fabricated over the pins to create a surgical template to assist the surgeon with the placement of the dental implants.

Several treatment plans were considered and discussed in detail with the patient. A conventional approach was offered that addressed the patient's needs through caries control, periodontal therapy, endodontic therapy, crown lengthening, and restorative procedures, including dowel and core foundations restored with full coverage restorations. This approach, in addition to being costly, was met with concerns by the patient based upon her restorative history. A second treatment option was given to extract teeth 34–36, maintain the osseous structure, and place two dental implants in sites 34 and 36 and restore them with a three-unit fixed dental prosthesis. While this may be viewed as an aggressive approach, the treatment was believed to have the best long-term prognosis, given the patient's dental history. When the cost was reviewed, the second option was also more feasible for the patient. Other conservative treatment options were also discussed and subsequently declined by the patient.

In the laboratory, the existing teeth were utilized to plan for implant positioning. A surgical template was fabricated to assist the surgeon in placing two immediate implants in sites 34 and 36 in an ideal restorative position, utilizing the available bone upon the extraction of the teeth (Higginbottom and coworkers, 1996).

At the surgical visit, teeth 34 – 36 were extracted, utilizing periotomes and forceps in an attempt to preserve osseous structure. Upon the removal of the teeth, the sockets were debrided with a curette and irrigated with NaCl solution. The proposed implant sites were examined to confirm that the cortical plates were intact. A surgical template was utilized to place implants in sites 34 – 36. Because the implants were to be positioned immediately, tapered effect implants (Straumann AG) were selected to maximize primary stability (Fig 4). Two healing caps were placed and a postoperative radiograph was taken (Figs 5 – 6). Postoperative instructions were given to the patient, and a one-week follow-up appointment was scheduled.

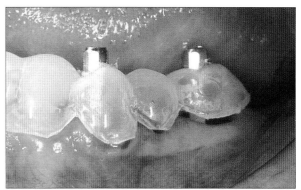

Fig 4   The surgical template in place, confirming the final position of the dental implants prior to the removal of the implant mount.

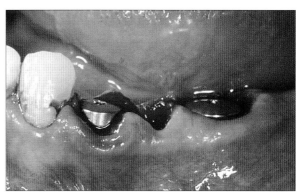

Fig 5   The dental implants with the healing caps in place.

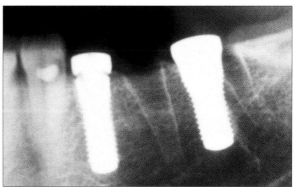

Fig 6   The postoperative periapical radiograph. Site 34: 4.1 x 12 mm RN, site 36: 4.8 x 12 mm WN.

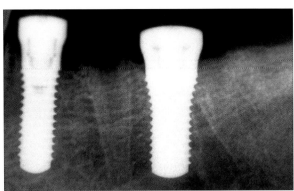

Fig 7   Periapical radiograph 6 weeks after implant placement.

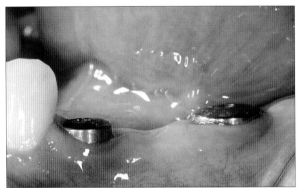

Fig 8   The lateral view of the implants 6 weeks after placement.

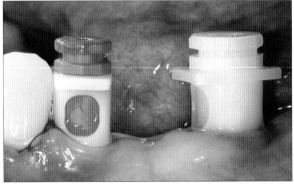

Fig 9   Lateral view of the impression caps and synOcta positioning cylinders in place.

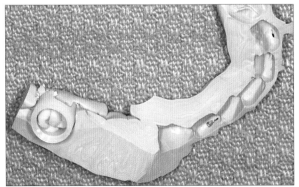

Fig 10   Jaw relation record with the impression cap in place.

At the one-week follow-up visit, the healing cap on the implant in site 34 was loose and was subsequently tightened with the SCS screwdriver. Six weeks after the placement of the dental implants, the patient returned for the final impression. A periapical radiograph was taken to view the extent of the socket healing (Fig 7). Prior to the final impression, a shade selection was made and photographed for laboratory communication. The healing caps were removed and impression caps and synOcta positioning cylinders were placed (Figs 8 – 9). A polyvinyl siloxane impression was made in addition to a jaw relation record. In clinical situations where implants are not bound by natural tooth stops distal to the most posterior implant, a second impression cap is captured within the jaw relation record to function as a third reference point for cast articulation (Fig 10). The healing caps were placed and the patient was scheduled for a delivery appointment.

In the laboratory, synOcta analogs were carefully snapped into the impression caps. A soft-tissue analog material was positioned around their collars and allowed to set (Fig 11). Excess tissue analog material was removed prior to pouring the impression in a low-expansion die stone. The master casts were articulated and definitive synOcta abutments were selected. The implants were placed in a parallel position that allowed cementable synOcta abutments to be utilized (Fig 12). The abutments were prepared with a twelve-fluted carbide bur to allow for a common path of insertion and adequate reduction for a metal-ceramic fixed dental prosthesis. A full-contour wax-up was created (Fig 13). The wax-up was cut back to allow for a uniform ceramic thickness (Fig 14). The wax pattern was sprued, invested, and cast in a high-noble ceramic alloy (Fig 15). Ceramic material was applied, and the prosthesis was completed (Figs 16 – 17).

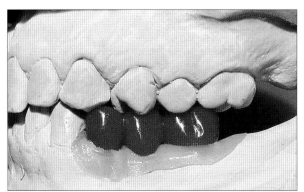
Fig 13   Lateral view of the full-contour wax-up.

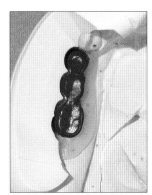
Fig 14   Occlusal view of the cutback with a putty matrix of the full-contour wax-up.

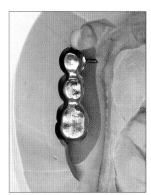
Fig 15   Occlusal view of the framework on the master cast with the matrix in place.

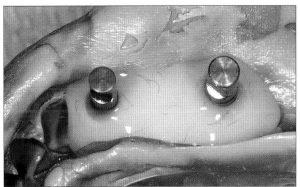
Fig 11   Intaglio surface of the final impression with synOcta analogs.

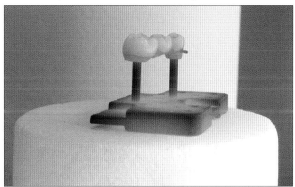
Fig 16   Ceramic firing.

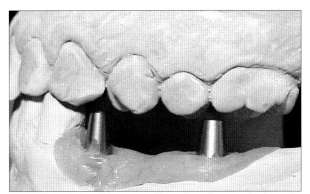
Fig 12   Lateral view of the cementable synOcta abutments in place prior to reduction.

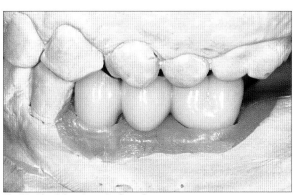
Fig 17   Fixed dental prosthesis on the master cast.

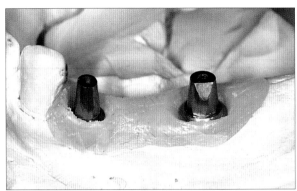

Fig 18   Prepared synOcta abutments on the master cast.

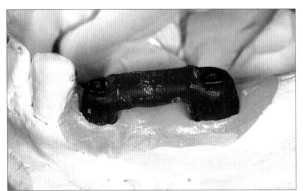

Fig 19   Acrylic resin index fabricated over the definitive synOcta abutments.

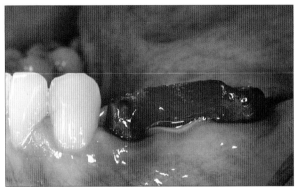

Fig 20   The transfer index placed on the dental implants.

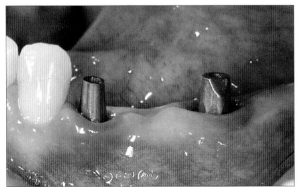

Fig 21   The definitive synOcta abutments prior to sealing with cotton and cavit.

Prior to returning the implant-supported fixed dental prosthesis, an abutment positioning or transfer index was fabricated to allow for the accurate placement of the synOcta abutments into the dental implants. In general, when multiple abutments that support a fixed dental prosthesis are prepared, their accurate placement into the implants may be difficult due to the multiple orientations that could occur. The fabrication of an acrylic resin transfer index that captures their orientation on the master cast allows for an accurate placement of the abutments into the oral cavity (Figs 18 – 19).

At the delivery appointment, the healing caps were removed and the implants cleansed with the air/water syringe. The transfer index (with the synOcta abutments in place) was placed into the implants (Fig 20). The abutments were hand-tightened and the fixed dental prosthesis was placed onto the implants. The fixed dental prosthesis was examined for accurate shade, passivity, and interproximal and occlusal contacts. Once the color and fit were confirmed, the synOcta abutments were tightened to 35 Ncm and sealed with cotton and cavit (Fig 21).

W. Martin, J. Ruskin

A definitive resin-modified cement was utilized to seat the restoration. Occlusion was refined and polished with diamond-impregnated burs (Figs 22 – 23). A periapical radiograph was taken, and the patient was scheduled for a follow-up appointment (Fig 24).

The patient was placed on a strict recall program and therapy was continued for other areas of concern. Follow-up pictures and radiographs were taken at four years (Figs 25 – 26).

Acknowledgments

Laboratory Procedures
Todd A. Fridrich – Definitive Dental Arts, Coralville, Iowa, USA.

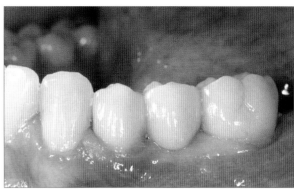

Fig 22   Lateral view of the fixed dental prosthesis.

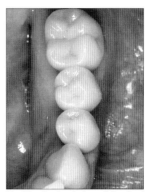

Fig 23   Occlusal view of the fixed dental prosthesis.

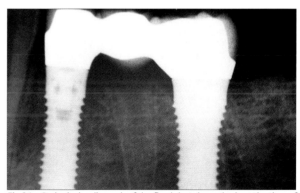

Fig 24   Periapical radiograph of the fixed dental prosthesis at the time of delivery.

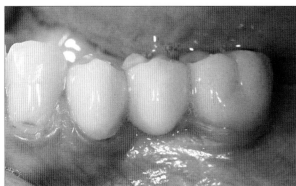

Fig 25   Lateral view of the fixed dental prosthesis at 4 years after implant placement.

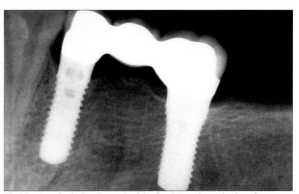

Fig 26   A periapical radiograph of the fixed dental prosthesis at four years.

4.3 Replacement of Multiple Teeth in a Partially Dentate Posterior Maxilla and Mandible with Fixed Dental Prostheses Using a Conventional Loading Protocol

G. O. Gallucci

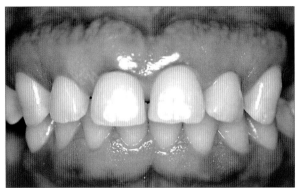

Fig 1 Frontal view in occlusion. The vertical dimension is consistently maintained by the remaining posterior and anterior teeth.

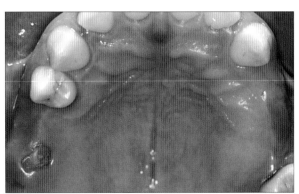

Fig 2 Maxillary occlusal view. The root fragment is clinically visible in the area of tooth 16.

In the summer of 2002, a 42-year-old female patient was referred to the University of Geneva for the replacement of posterior maxillary and mandibular missing or non-restorable teeth. The patient's medical history revealed no significant findings, and she was in good general health. Her dental history included recurrent decay that led to the loss of several posterior teeth. The patient showed no history of periodontal disease.

At the extraoral examination, the patient presented normal physiognomy with normal facial and lip support and homogenous distribution of the facial thirds. At full smiling, the patient displayed an average lip line, and a tooth gap was slightly visible in the left maxilla. Small diastemas were present between the anterior maxillary teeth (Fig 1).

The patient's chief complaint was "discomfort when chewing and speaking," which called for the replacement of the posterior missing teeth. The patient had no esthetic concerns regarding her current dental status. The patient ruled out a removable solution and requested a fixed restoration.

At the intraoral evaluation, the patient presented with multi-tooth gaps in the posterior maxilla and the right posterior mandible. The missing teeth were recorded as follows: 17, 16, 15, 24, 25, 26, 37, 45, 46, and 47. In the area of tooth 16, a residual root fragment resulting from an incomplete tooth extraction was clinically visible (Fig 2).

Radiographic analysis revealed the recent extraction of tooth 45. This finding became important to the treatment planning for implant placement.

Radiographically, the residual root fragment appeared to be small and sequestered within the edentulous mucosa without any signs of acute inflammation. The radiological aspect of the partial dentition displayed three similar multi-tooth gaps. The maxillary ridges presented adequate coronoapical dimension for implant placement. A similar situation was observed in the mandible, where the inferior alveolar nerve was located rather apically, leaving enough space for a straightforward implant placement (Fig 3). Since the clinical evaluation revealed good orofacial dimension, the orthopanoramic radiograph and mounted diagnostic casts were judged to be sufficient for diagnostic and treatment-planning purposes.

The treatment plan considered 3 three-unit implant-supported restorations to restore the maxillary right and left posterior sectors, as well as the mandibular right posterior zone. The vertical dimension of occlusion and occlusal contacts were stable at centric relation. The dimensions of the multi-tooth gaps were homogenous and presented a correct mesiodistal dimension for the allocation of three prosthetic units. Based on these diagnostic elements, implant placement was performed with two implants per multi-tooth gap (Fig 4).

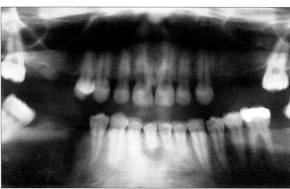

Fig 3   Panoramic radiograph displaying enough bone height. The residual root fragment and the post-extraction area 45 were issues to be considered for the treatment planning.

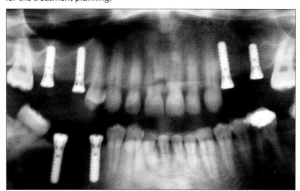

Fig 4   Post-surgical radiograph. The prosthetics-driven implant allocation and distribution ensured the fabrication of 3 three-unit fixed dental prostheses.

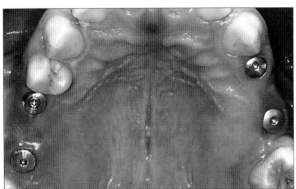

Fig 5   Clinical status of maxillary implants after 4 months of non-functional healing.

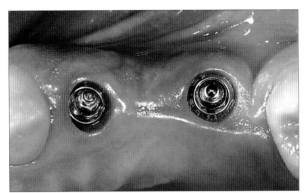

Fig 6   Close-up view of implants at sites 24 and 26, showing the healing status of the maxillary peri-implant mucosa.

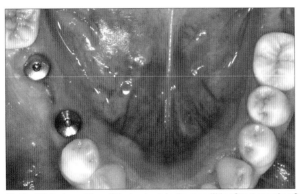

Fig 7   Clinical condition of the implants in the mandible after 4 months of undisturbed healing.

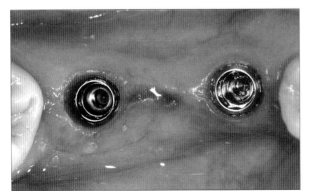

Fig 8   Close-up view of the implants in sites 45 and 47, showing the healing status of the mandibular peri-implant soft tissue after the removal of the healing caps.

Six Straumann Standard Plus implants (endosteal diameter, 4.1 mm; length, 12 mm (sites 15, 24, 45, 47) and 10 mm (sites 17, 26); Regular Neck prosthetic platform, 4.8 mm) were placed. Primary stability was achieved with all implants, and flaps were repositioned in a non-submerged surgical approach. In order to enhance the esthetic appearance of the edentulous ridge, a lateral bone augmentation was performed simultaneously to the implant placement. During the healing phase, the patient was given a soft toothbrush and instructions for implant maintenance with chlorhexidine mouthwash during the first week.

After a healing period of 4 months, the healing caps were removed and the soft tissue status was assessed (Figs 5 – 8).

A provisional phase was considered to be not essential in this particular case. The overall esthetic appearance was not compromised, and the vertical dimension of the occlusion was stable. Based on these parameters, the decision was made to proceed with the final restoration and to shorten the total treatment time.

Therefore, final impressions were made. Final upper and lower impressions were made at the implant level using two different kinds of impression copings. In the maxilla, screw-on impression copings were used due to the slightly deeper placement of the implants (Fig 9). In the mandible, the snap-on impression approach was selected according to a more superficial implant placement and a slightly thinner peri-implant mucosa (Fig 10).

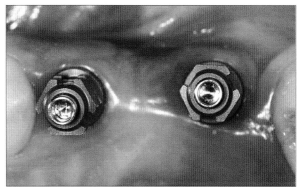

Fig 9   Prior to taking the implant-level impression at sites 24 and 26. Screw-on impression caps were selected for the maxillary open-tray final impression.

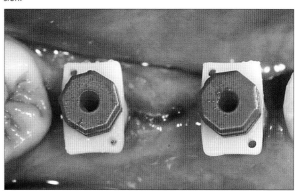

Fig 10   Prior to taking the implant-level impression of the implants in the mandible. Snap-on impression caps were selected for the closed-tray final impression.

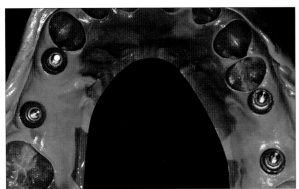

Fig 11   Impression with screw-on synOcta impression copings. Final maxillary open-tray impression.

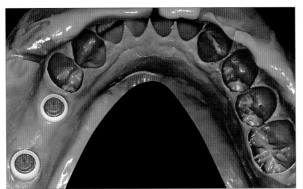

Fig 12   Impression with snap-on synOcta impression copings. Final mandibular closed-tray impression.

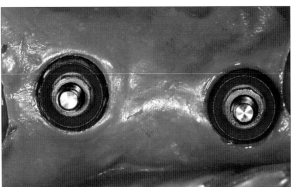

Fig 13   Maxillary final impression. Close-up view of screw-on copings.

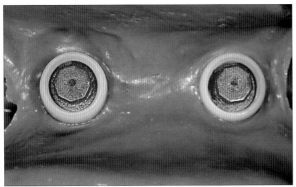

Fig 14   Mandibular impression. Close-up view of snap-on copings.

After the interarch relationship was recorded, healing caps were tightened back onto the implants and the patient was rescheduled for the frameworks try-in one week later.

The different synOcta impression copings offered the same versatility at the time of fabricating the master cast (Figs 11 – 12). In the retrieved impression trays, the copings provided a stable fit for the implant analogs. Once the analogs were connected to the impression copings, the implant location was reproduced along with the position of the antirotational internal octagon (Figs 13 – 14).

The selection of the definitive abutments was completed once the master casts, including the implant analogs, were fabricated and articulated (Fig 15). The implant-level impression offered the possibility of selecting the best suitable abutments on the mounted casts. In this particular case, five 4-mm solid abutments and an angled synOcta abutment were used according to the planned restorations and the occlusal relationship.

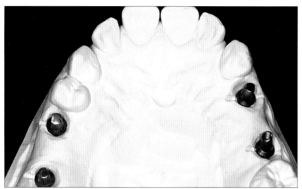

Fig 15   Maxillary master cast. Definitive abutments have been selected and used during the entire fabrication process of the fixed dental prosthesis before definitive transfer to the patient's mouth.

Plastic copings (for the fixed dental prosthesis, FDP) and a synOcta coping (for the angled abutment) were used for the fabrication of the frameworks. The frameworks were fabricated directly onto the definitive abutments (Figs 16 – 17). In the areas where 4-mm solid abutments were used, the internal configuration of the copings (for FDP) resulted in a framework that ensured the definitive abutments could be transferred from the cast to the patient's mouth. This would allow for the passive seating of the FDP (Figs 18 – 21).

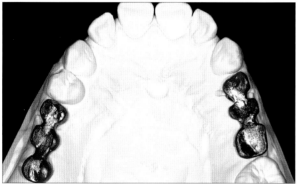

Fig 16   Maxillary frameworks.

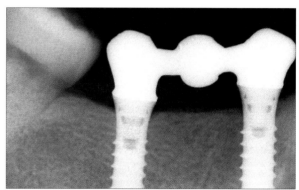

Fig 19   Radiographic assessment of the marginal adaptation of the mandibular framework.

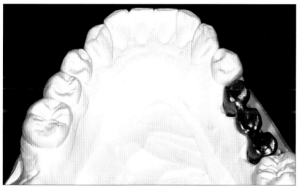

Fig 17   Mandibular framework.

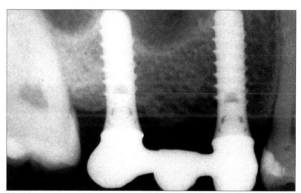

Fig 20   Radiographic assessment of the marginal adaptation of the right maxillary framework.

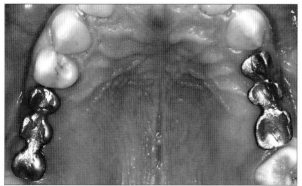

Fig 18   Maxillary frameworks try-in.

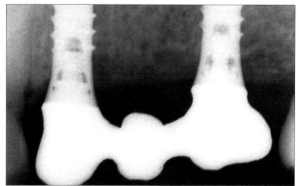

Fig 21   Radiographic assessment of the marginal adaptation of the left maxillary framework.

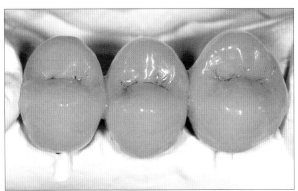

Fig 22   Definitive rehabilitation on the master cast.

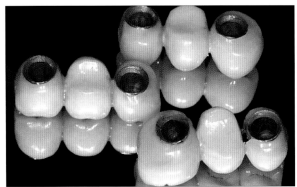

Fig 23   Internal view of the 3 three-unit FDPs.

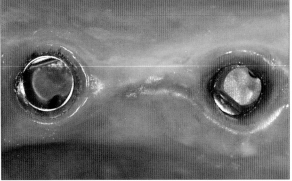

Fig 24   Sandblasted abutments were tightened to 35 Ncm.

Following the metal frameworks try-in and before proceeding with the ceramic veneer, the occlusal relationship was verified. The ceramic work was then completed using a stratification technique, and the prostheses were glazed to achieve a natural-looking appearance (Figs 22 – 23).

At delivery, the healing abutments were removed and the definitive abutments were tightened to 35 Ncm. At this stage, none of the six implants rotated and the patient manifested no discomfort. Due to the abridged abutment length (4 mm), the solid abutments were sandblasted to improve mechanical retention (Fig 24). After an assessment of the seating and the pressure of the proximal contact areas, occlusal adjustment was undertaken, and the restoration was cemented (Figs 25 – 26).

This case resulted in a conventional loading approach with definitive restorations, avoiding a provisional phase. The implant-supported restorations were initially cemented with provisional cement and, after a reasonable follow-up period, a dual-cure adhesive agent was used for the final cementation.

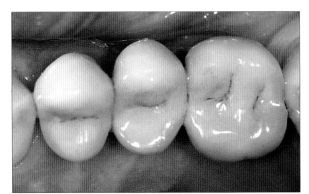

Fig 25   Occlusal view of the left maxillary implant-supported FDP.

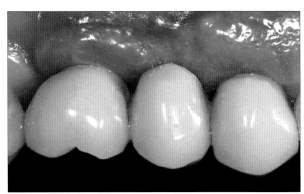

Fig 26   Lateral view of the maxillary left implant-supported FDP after cementation.

A panoramic radiograph was then taken to assess the final treatment outcome (Fig 27).

The patient received maintenance instructions and was followed-up by the dental hygienist every three months during the first year. After that, she was referred to the regular recall system at the Student Clinic, University of Geneva.

At the 2-year follow-up, the patient presented a satisfactory clinical status (Figs 28 – 31).

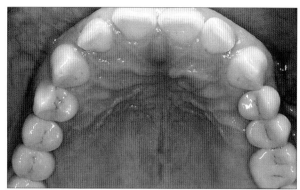

Fig 28   Maxillary occlusal view at 2-year follow-up.

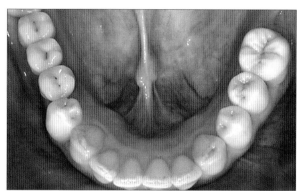

Fig 29   2-year follow-up, mandibular view.

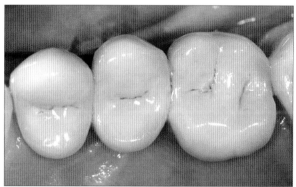

Fig 30   Close-up view of the maxillary right FDP at the 2-year follow-up.

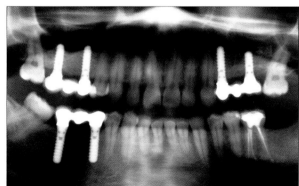

Fig 27   Final radiograph of the outcome.

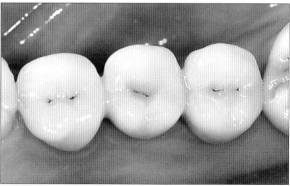

Fig 31   Close-up view of the mandibular FDP at the 2-year follow-up.

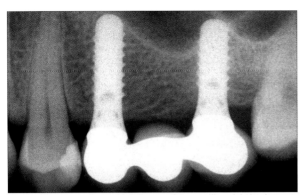

Fig 32   Two-year radiographic follow-up of the maxillary right implant-supported FDP.

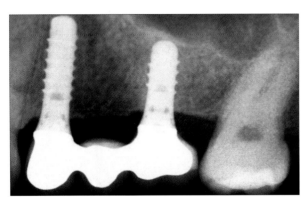

Fig 33   Two-year radiographic follow-up of the maxillary left implant-supported FDP.

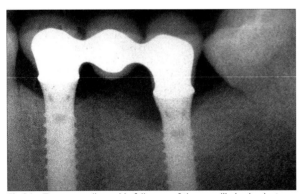

Fig 34   Two-year radiographic follow-up of the mandibular implant-supported FDP.

At the radiographic evaluation, optimal conditions at the peri-implant bone level were observed (Figs 32 – 34).

Acknowledgments

Surgical Procedures
Dr. Stéphane Pessotto – University of Geneva, Department of Stomatology and Oral Surgery.

Laboratory Procedures
Michel Bertossa – CDT, University of Geneva, Department of Fixed Prosthodontics.

4.4 Replacement of Multiple Teeth in a Partially Dentate Posterior Maxilla with a Fixed Dental Prosthesis and a Crown Using Conventional Loading Protocols

F. Higginbottom, T. Wilson

This 65-year-old female patient presented for implant-based restoration of the maxillary posterior region (25 – 27). Although this patient was free of medical compromise, her treatment was associated with several modifying factors.

She had been a patient of record in the practice for more than twenty years. Her initial treatment included extraction of the failing maxillary left first molar (Fig 1), and restoration with a fixed dental prosthesis (25 – 27) and crown (24). At the time of initial restoration, implants were not considered appropriate options for the replacement of single posterior teeth.

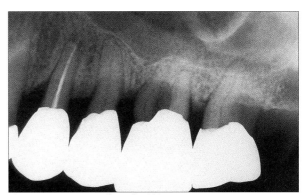

Fig 1   Pre-treatment radiograph, 1982.

The fixed dental prosthesis ultimately failed as a result of recurrent dental caries (Fig 2). Although the patient was provided with an implant-based treatment option for the re-treatment, this was declined because of the need for sinus elevation. A new tooth-supported fixed dental prosthesis was therefore fabricated. After approximately 7 years, the new prosthesis also failed, resulting in the loss of both abutment teeth.

The patient accepted a new treatment plan, which included sinus elevation and ridge augmentation before implant placement. The grafts were allowed to heal for 6 months prior to implant placement.

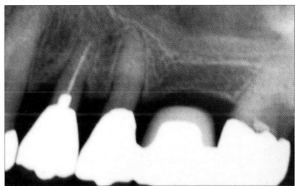

Fig 2   Radiograph of the initial FDP.

Treatment was complicated by several modifying factors. These included bruxism, the absence of adequate anterior guidance, the less than favorable crown to implant ratios and the presence of type 4 bone.

Modifying factors:

- Bruxism
- Minimal anterior guidance
- Unfavorable crown-to-implant ratio
- Type 4 bone

These factors influenced the treatment options given to the patient. The available treatment choices were: doing nothing, placing a removable partial prosthesis, or placing dental implants and fixed dental prostheses. The patient choose the implant-based treatment option, and she was scheduled for sinus and ridge augmentation. A provisional removable partial prosthesis was fabricated for limited wear during the healing period. After 6 months of healing, the placement of three implants was planned (25: endosteal diameter, 4.1 mm; length, 10 mm; Regular Neck platform, 4.8 mm; 27: endosteal diameter, 4.8 mm; length, 8 mm; Regular Neck platform, 4.8 mm − all Standard Plus implants) (Fig 3), and undertaken (Fig 4).

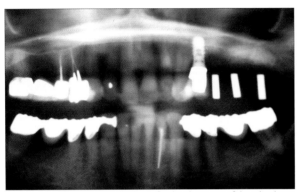

Fig 3   Treatment planning alignment for the placement of three implants.

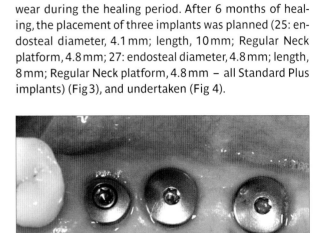

Fig 6   Occlusal view of the implants after 12 weeks of healing.

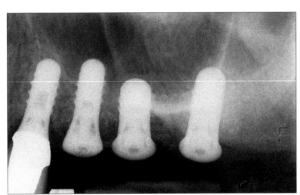

Fig 4   Radiograph of implants placed in sinus graft (12 weeks).

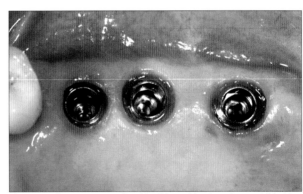

Fig 7   Healing caps removed and healthy peri-implant tissues visible. Note the relatively flat gingival contour, allowing for a cemented restoration.

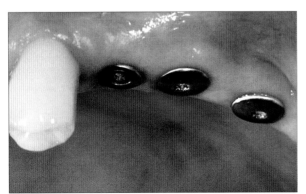

Fig 5   Clinical appearance of the implants in good position after 12 weeks of healing.

After twelve weeks of healing, restorative procedures began with impressions and provisional restorations (Figs 5 – 7).

Definitive impressions were made using screw-on synOcta impression copings (Figs 8 – 9).

The implants were provisionalized using 4-mm solid abutments and an autopolymerizing resin fixed dental prosthesis (Figs 10 – 11).

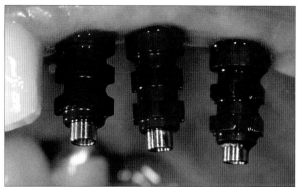

Fig 8   Screw-on synOcta impression copings seated for a open-tray impression.

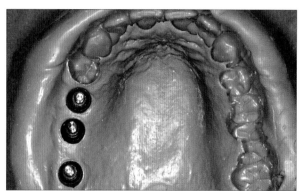

Fig 9   Definitive impression taken with polyvinyl impression material.

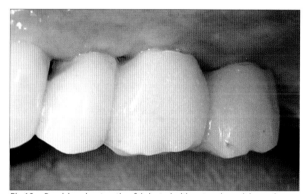

Fig 10   Provisional restoration fabricated with autopolymerizing resin over 4-mm solid abutments.

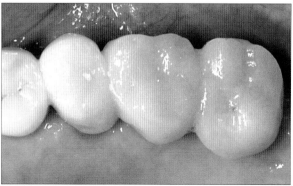

Fig 11   Occlusal view of the splinted provisional restoration.

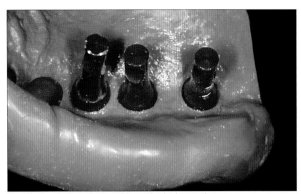

Fig 12   Implant analogs positioned in the impression.

Due to the modifying factors identified in the introduction, it was decided to splint the implants together with one fixed prosthesis. However, this presented a problem due to the angulation differences between the implants. There were several options for solving the angulation problem. Solid abutments could be prepared in the mouth. Custom abutments could be used, but the implants were considered too shallow for this option. Angled abutments presented the third and most viable choice. The angled abutments were selected in the laboratory using the Straumann prosthetic planning kit (Figs 12 – 15) .

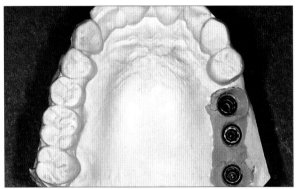

Fig 13   Master cast poured, with soft tissue analog adapted around the implant analog shoulders.

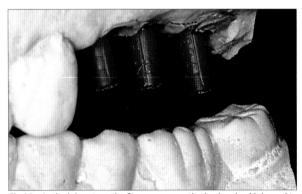

Fig 14   In the laboratory, the Straumann prosthetic planning kit is used to select the appropriate angled abutment.

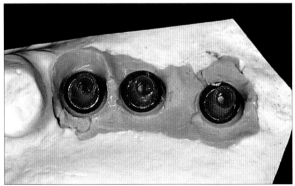

Fig 15   Occlusal view of the planning abutments selected, illustrating the parallelism.

After the selection of the appropriate abutments, a metal framework was constructed and returned for the verification of passivity in the mouth (Figs 16 – 20).

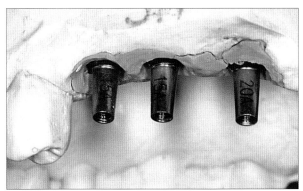

Fig 16 Two 15A and one 20A synOcta angled abutments are selected and seated on the master cast.

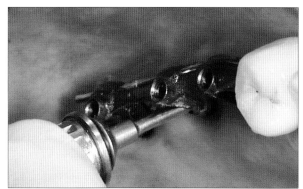

Fig 19 Angled abutments seated as a unit. The index will be removed for the framework try-in.

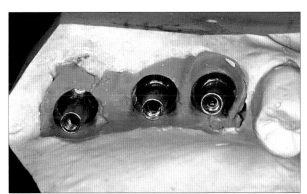

Fig 17 Occlusal view of the abutments selected. A framework will be fabricated for verification in the mouth.

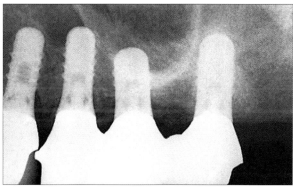

Fig 20 Radiographic view of the framework in place. The radiograph inclination was not appropriate for assessment of the restoration-implant interface (lack of thread visibility indicates less than ideal parallelism). The fit was satisfactory both visibly and by tactile senses.

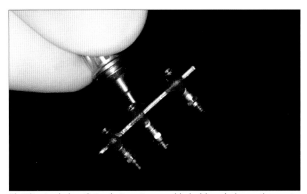

Fig 18 Angled synOcta abutments assembled with an index on the master cast to carry to the mouth in one piece.

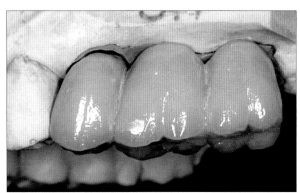
Fig 21   Completed metal-ceramic restoration.

After the verification of the articulation records, the framework was returned to the laboratory for ceramic application (Figs 21 – 23).

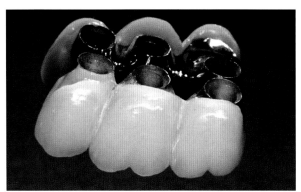
Fig 22   Completed metal-ceramic restoration.

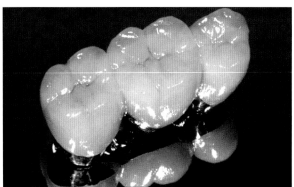
Fig 23   Completed metal-ceramic restoration.

The metal-ceramic fixed dental prosthesis was fitted and the occlusion adjusted. The restoration was seated with provisional cement, which would allow for removal, if necessary (Figs 24 – 29).

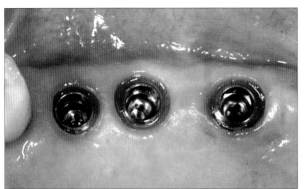

Fig 24   Provisional restoration removed, showing stable and nicely shaped peri-implant soft tissues.

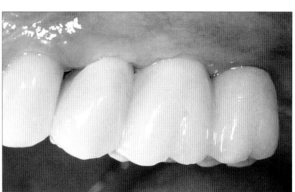

Fig 27   Final restoration seated.

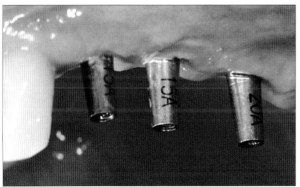

Fig 25   Angled synOcta abutments seated and torqued to 35 Ncm.

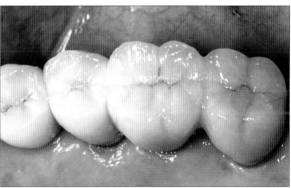

Fig 28   Occlusal view of final restoration.

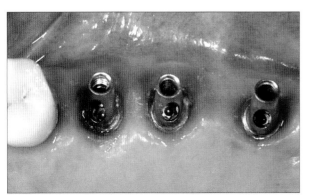

Fig 26   Angled synOcta abutments seated and torqued to 35 Ncm.

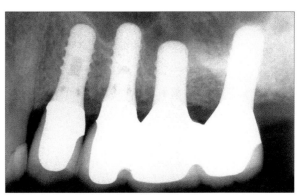

Fig 29   Radiograph at insertion of final restoration.

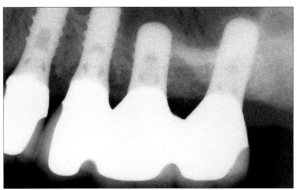

Fig 30   Five-year recall radiograph.

After two weeks, the patient returned for a post-insertion evaluation and the insertion of a habit appliance. The patient has had an uneventful follow-up period of over five years (Fig 30).

Acknowledgments

Laboratory Procedures
Jeff Singler

4.5 Replacement of Multiple Teeth in a Partially Dentate Posterior Maxilla with Crowns Using a Conventional Loading Protocol

G. S. Solnit, M. Kaufman

In 2004, an 84-year-old female patient presented at our practice with a hopeless prognosis for her maxillary right first and second premolars. These teeth were supporting a three-unit fixed dental prosthesis and had a cantilevered pontic replacing the first molar. Both teeth had combined endodontic and periodontal lesions, with significant bone loss in the area. The patient also had a large maxillary sinus apical to the first molar site (Fig 1).

The patient presented with normal facial form and upon normal smiling, she displayed the affected area. She reported mobility and pain with mastication. The fixed dental prosthesis displayed severe mobility and could be depressed into the alveolar sockets. Exudate was evident around both abutments. There were no significant medical problems reported and the patient reported taking no medications.

Both teeth were extracted and the existing prosthesis removed, and the alveolar sockets were grafted with autogenous bone and bone substitute material mixed together. The maxillary sinus was also grafted in the same fashion. The patient did not wear an interim prosthesis for two weeks. After two weeks, an interim removable partial denture was delivered and adjusted so that no pressure was exerted over the grafted areas. The denture was relined with a soft liner and checked every three to four weeks. The liner was changed as needed and each time, the area was checked carefully to make sure there was no pressure over the grafted sites. The grafts were allowed to heal undisturbed for three months.

After three months of healing, three Straumann implants were placed in the first premolar, second premolar, and first molar positions, utilizing a surgical template. Implants with a Regular Neck prosthetic platform were placed in the premolar positions and an implant with a Wide Neck prosthetic platform was placed in the molar site. The interim denture was again relieved and checked to make sure no pressure was exerted over the implants. The implants were allowed to heal for six weeks undisturbed.

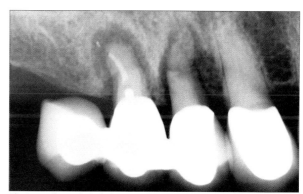

Fig 1   Radiograph depicting the condition of the existing fixed dental prosthesis at consultation.

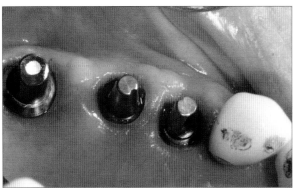

Fig 2   Occlusal view of the solid abutments in place. Note the correct mesial/distal and buccal/lingual positioning of the implants. A slight reduction of the solid abutment in the molar site provided more clearance for restorative materials.

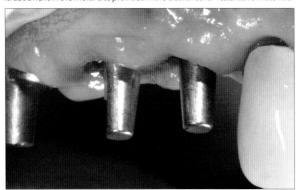

Fig 3   Buccal view of the solid abutments in place. Note the shallow depth of the implant placement, making the cemented approach a more acceptable restorative option.

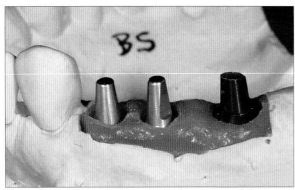

Fig 4   The master cast with the analogs in place and the soft tissue mask. Note the reduction on the analog in the molar site, which was recorded using a plastic coping.

After conventional healing (4 months) was complete, three 5.5-mm solid abutments were placed and torqued to 35 Ncm. Because of the acceptable angulation and shallow placement of the implants, the cemented approach for the final restorations was indicated. The 5.5-mm solid abutments were appropriate for adequate retention of the final restorations. They also allowed space for acceptable metal ceramic restorations. The solid abutment in the molar region was reduced slightly to provide a little more space. This was considered a better alternative than placing a 4.0-mm abutment, which may have had inadequate retention for the final restoration (Figs 2 – 3). A plastic reduction coping was fabricated and provided to the laboratory.

Standard impression procedures were followed, utilizing the snap-on impression components. An impression was made using a custom tray and a polyvinyl siloxane impression material. The master cast was poured in a low expansion dental stone. A soft tissue mask was fabricated over the analogs to simulate the emergence of the surrounding soft tissue. Tissue expansion was not necessary, as the implants were of the appropriate emergence diameter and the implants were placed at the appropriate depth (Fig 4).

The final metal-ceramic restorations were fabricated as individual units. Proximal contacts were carefully adjusted on the master cast to ensure tight contacts and the completely passive seating of the restorations (Fig 5).

The restorations were tried into the patient's mouth to verify passive fit with a silicone fit checking material. Proximal contacts were verified with mylar shimstock and dental floss. Extreme care must be taken during the seating of individual restorations on implants. It is imperative that a silicone medium is utilized to assess the complete seating of the restorations because proximal contacts can prevent seating completely. Detrimental forces to the implants are also possible.

Once the complete seating of the restorations was established, they were temporarily cemented in position with the same silicone medium. The occlusion was checked to ensure centric contacts and adequate clearance during excursive movements with articulating paper (Fig 6).

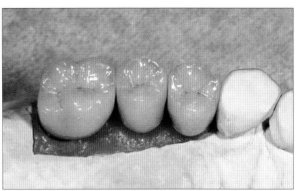

Fig 5 The final individual metal-ceramic restorations on the master cast. All proximal contacts were carefully adjusted to ensure adequate contact and the passive seating of the restorations.

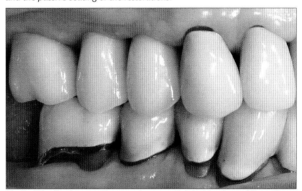

Fig 6 The final restorations are temporarily luted to place with a silicone medium. The occlusion can then be checked to ensure appropriate centric contacts and proper disclusion during excursive movements.

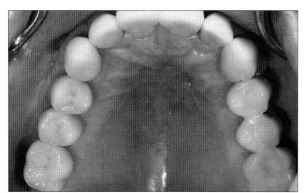

Fig 7   Occlusal view of the final restorations.

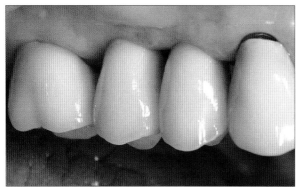

Fig 8   Buccal view of the final restorations.

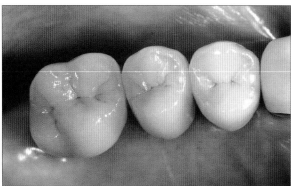

Fig 9   Occlusal view of the final restorations. Note the acceptable proximal contacts between the individual restorations.

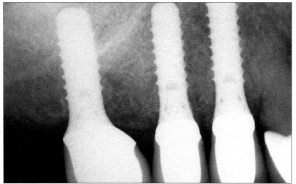

Fig 10   Periapical radiograph depicting the passive fit of the restorations and good bone-to-implant contact surrounding all three implants.

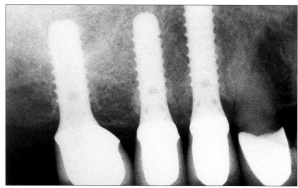

Fig 11   Radiograph taken at the three year follow-up.

Once the occlusion was verified, the final restorations were luted to place with a resin-reinforced glass-ionomer cement. A thin layer of cement was applied and the excess was carefully removed while the patient was fully anesthetized (Figs 7 – 9). A periapical radiograph was taken to assess the final outcome of treatment (Fig 10). A periapical radiograph was taken once again at the three-year follow-up (Fig. 11).

Acknowledgments

Laboratory Procedures
Tim Ide

4.6 Replacement of Two Teeth in a Partially Dentate Posterior Maxilla with a Fixed Dental Prosthesis Using a Conventional Loading Protocol

U. Belser, D. Buser

In September of 1995, a 64-year-old female patient presented to our clinic with a distally shortened arch in the left maxilla and the desire for a fixed rehabilitation. The patient's medical history did not reveal any major issues, and she did not take any significant medication. She was a non-smoker and did not report any allergies. The patient wished to restore her chewing function on the left side, which was severely compromised due to the missing teeth 25, 26, and 27. The antagonistic lower teeth were present and in acceptable condition.

A decision was made together with the patient to place two implants according to a staged protocol at sites 25 and 26 (25: Straumann Standard implant, endosteal diameter, 4.1 mm; length, 12 mm; Regular Neck prosthetic platform, 4.8 mm; 26: Straumann Standard implant, endosteal diameter, 4.8 mm; length, 10 mm; Regular Neck prosthetic platform, 4.8 mm), after a sinus-grafting procedure. Sinus grafting was necessary to establish adequate bone volume for stable implant placement, due to the insufficient bone height at the future implantation sites (Fig 1). The patient gave her informed consent that – as this was the standard of care at that time – a healing period of at least 6 months would be utilized after the sinus-grafting procedure before the implants could be placed. Furthermore, under these conditions, i.e. implants inserted into grafted bone, a conventional loading protocol comprising 3 months of healing prior to restoration represented the standard procedure.

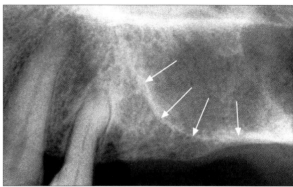

Fig 1 Radiograph of the posterior region of the left maxilla. The wide-stretching maxillary sinus at sites 25 – 27 and the resulting lack of vertical bone height in this region are clearly visible. For stable implant anchorage, a sinus-grafting procedure was considered indispensable.

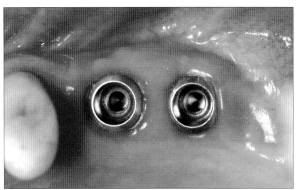

Fig 2 Implants 25 and 26 after the removal of the healing caps, 12 weeks after the implant placement. Note the superficial location of the implant shoulders and the related inflammation-free peri-implant mucosa.

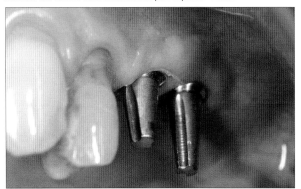

Fig 3 The situation 12 weeks after implant placement, before impression-taking, in view of the fabrication of a provisional restoration. Two solid abutments have been inserted.

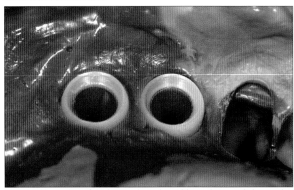

Fig 4 Close-up view of the impression taken with an elastomeric impression material. The two implant shoulders have been picked up by means of self-anchoring injection-molded impression caps.

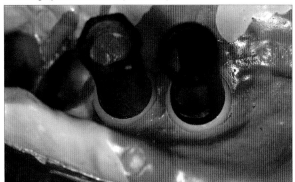

Fig 5 The impression with the shoulder analogs in place, before the insertion of the reinforcement pins.

At the time of implant placement, i.e. 8 months after the anterior sinus-grafting procedure, good primary stability was achieved. Subsequent to implant surgery, the implants were allowed to heal for 12 weeks.

At the time of the removal of the healing caps 12 weeks after implant placement, the mucosa presented healthy and free from bleeding on probing (Fig 2). The implants were well integrated and revealed ankylotic stability, so the decision was made to make an impression for loading with a provisional restoration, according to a conventional loading protocol (Ganeles and Wismeijer, 2004).

Two solid abutments, 5.5 mm and 7.0 mm in length, were secured on the implants at a torque of 35 Ncm – note both the superficial implant shoulder location, compatible with cemented restorations, and the optimal implants axis and parallelism (Fig 3). Then, an impression was taken to generate a master cast (Fig 4).

Subsequent to impression-making, two self-anchoring plastic shoulder analogs were positioned on the impression caps (Fig 5). Before pouring the cast, reinforcement pins were inserted. In 1996, integral implant analogs were not yet available, so at that time, this approach was the preferred one.

Subsequently, the cast was poured, with the cervical portions of the shoulder analogs representing the implant shoulders (Fig 6).

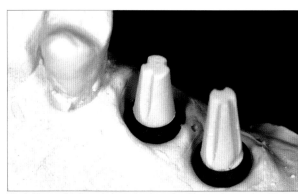

Fig 6 The prefabricated plastic implant shoulder analogs and solid abutments, represented in stone in sites 25 and 26.

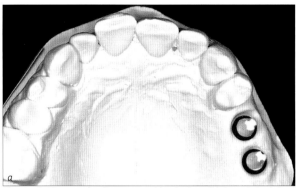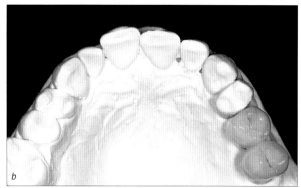

Figs 7a – b   The completed cast, comprising both prefabricated plastic implant shoulder analogs and solid abutments, represented in stone in sites 25 and 26, and the splinted, cementable provisional implant crowns before delivery, on the cast.

In the dental laboratory, a splinted provisional restoration was fabricated from acrylic resin (Figs 7 – 8). This was cemented to the solid abutments in the patient's mouth two weeks after impression-making (Figs 9a – b). The provisional restoration was loaded according to a conventional loading protocol.

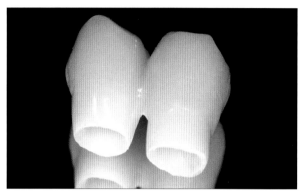

Fig 8   The cementable provisional implant crowns in close-up view.

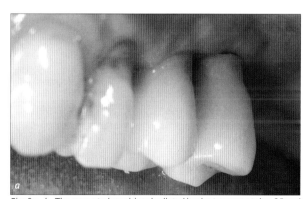

Figs 9a – b   The cemented provisional splinted implant crowns at sites 25 and 26 in the patient's mouth at about 14 weeks after implant placement, buccal and occlusal views, conventionally loaded.

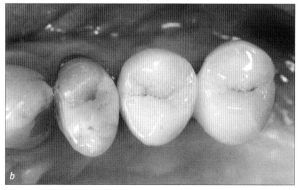

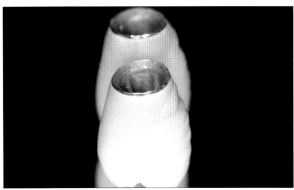

Fig 10 Close-up view of the two-unit splinted cementable metal-ceramic FDP before delivery. Note the flat emergence profile of the restoration.

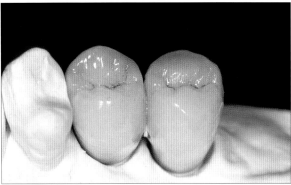

Fig 11 The splinted cementable metal-ceramic FDP on the master cast.

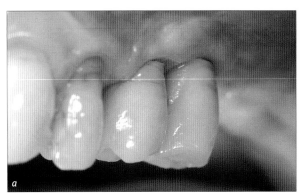

Figs 12a – b The final restoration in the patient's mouth after cementation, labial and occlusal aspects.

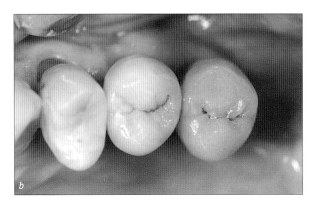

This timing permitted the patient to become accustomed with the fixed implant prosthesis and to approve the proposed design for the final prosthesis.

The provisional restoration remained in situ for eight weeks. About 10 weeks after the patient's first prosthodontic visit to our clinic, a final impression was made for the fabrication of the final restoration.

A two-unit splinted metal-ceramic fixed dental prosthesis (FPD) was fabricated in the dental laboratory. Again, a cemented design was chosen (Figs 10 – 11).

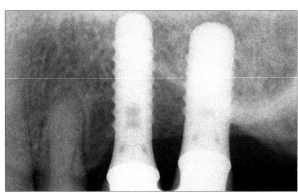

Fig 13 The periapical radiograph, taken after the cementation of the final restoration at about 15 weeks after the patient's first visit to our clinic, confirms normal peri-implant bone structures as well as the precise seating of the suprastructure on the implants.

Eleven years later, the conventionally loaded implants are still functioning successfully (Figs 14 – 15).

Meanwhile, tooth 24 received endodontic treatment and a metal-ceramic crown.

Concluding Remarks (Epicrisis):

In retrospect, both the number and location of the implants and the choice of splinting of the respective implants should be questioned.

First, the original status of tooth 24 (extremely short root) would probably have justified its extraction in the scope of a more general treatment plan addressing the distally shortened left maxillary arch. In fact, tooth 24 later required root-canal therapy and a subsequent restoration with a metal-ceramic crown, considerably increasing treatment costs and still representing a limited prognosis. In other words, its extraction would have allowed either a reconstructive solution based on implants in sites 24 and 25, comprising a distally cantilevered unit, or implants in sites 24 and 26, restored with a three-unit fixed dental prosthesis, comprising a central pontic. The first solution would have permitted the avoidance of a sinus grafting procedure and thus led to a significantly less invasive overall treatment.

Second, the splinting of the two implants in 25 and 26 may not have been necessary. There is no strong evidence in the current literature that indicates that implants placed in grafted bone require splinting. One should keep in mind, however, that single implant restorations offer the advantage of superior marginal fidelity as well as the ease of an eventual reintervention. Furthermore, they facilitate routine oral hygiene measures.

Acknowledgments

Laboratory Procedures
Alwin Schönenberger – Master Dental Technician, Glattbrugg, Switzerland.

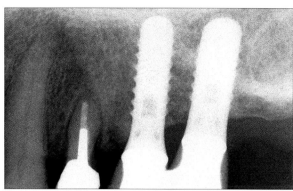

Fig 14 Radiologic follow-up 11 years after implant placement. The peri-implant bone is stable.

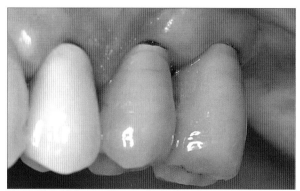

Fig 15 Clinical follow-up 11 years after implant placement.

Single-Tooth Gaps in the Posterior Maxilla or Mandible

4.7 Replacement of a Maxillary Left Second Premolar Using an Immediate Restoration Protocol

D. Morton, J. Ruskin

In June 2002, a healthy and cooperative 42-year-old female patient was referred for consultation and for the treatment of a fractured maxillary left second premolar (Fig 1).

The patient reported an uncomplicated medical history, significant only for seasonal allergies. She had been in the continuous care of a general dental practitioner at the University of Florida College of Dentistry for more than ten years, her recent dental history being restricted to routine operative dentistry and periodontal maintenance. Her plaque control and gingival health was considered for the most part to be excellent, and no intraoral periodontal probing depths exceeded 3 mm.

Her esthetic demands were considered moderate to high, and she displayed a high smile line (Fig 2). Intraoral examination revealed a Class I malocclusion, characterized by minor tooth misalignment and midline disharmony, for which orthodontic therapy was recommended and rejected (Figs 3 – 4). Her gingival biotype was considered medium to thick.

The maxillary second premolar (25) had previously been restored with an MOD amalgam restoration, and it displayed a fracture of the palatal cusp that extended into the periodontal attachment. The treatment options included:

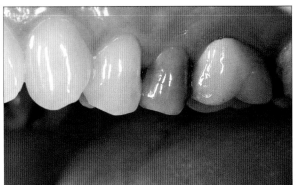

Fig 1 Pre-treatment lateral view of maxillary second premolar (25).

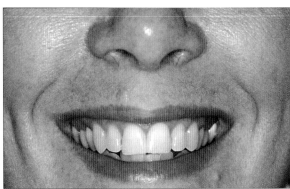

Fig 2 Pre-treatment smile.

- Option 1: Nonsurgical endodontic treatment and tooth elongation to expose healthy tooth structure on the palatal aspect, to be followed by a conventional foundation and metal-ceramic restoration.
- Option 2: Removal of the tooth, placement of an endosseous implant and, subsequent to healing, restoration with a metal-ceramic crown.

Endodontic and periodontic consultations were obtained. Treatment option 1 was considered to be compromised by the length and dimension of the radicular portion of the tooth and the small mesiodistal tooth width. Although the tooth could have been restored, as noted in treatment option 1, the patient ultimately chose option 2 as a simplified and cost-effective treatment alternative. The site was considered to be favorable for immediate (Type 1; Hammerle and coworkers, 2004) implant placement and immediate restoration (Cochran and coworkers, 2004) (provisional restoration out of contact with the opposing dentition).

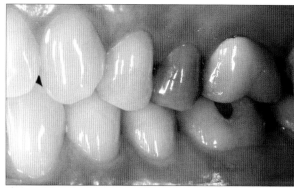
Fig 3 Pre-treatment lateral view. Maximum intercuspation.

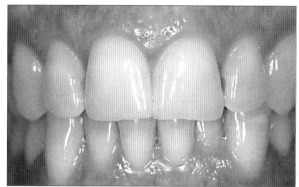
Fig 4 Anterior view and tissue biotype.

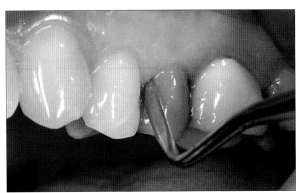

Fig 5   Minimally traumatic periotome extraction of tooth 25.

The tooth was extracted with periotomes to minimize trauma to the surrounding bone and soft tissues (Fig 5). A Straumann Tapered Effect implant (endosteal diameter, 4.1 mm; length, 10 mm, Regular Neck prosthetic platform, 4.8 mm) was immediately placed according to a restoration-driven protocol utilizing surgical templates, in order to ensure appropriate three-dimensional positioning (Figs 6 – 7).

Subsequent to implant placement, a radiograph was obtained to confirm implant position, and the implant stability was confirmed using resonance frequency analysis (Figs 8 – 9).

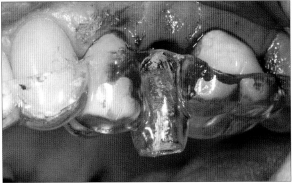

Fig 6   Sleeve template to guide mesiodistal and orofacial implant position.

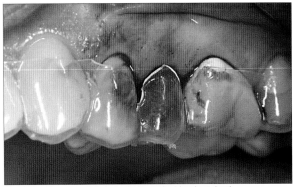

Fig 7   Vacuform template to indicate desired implant depth.

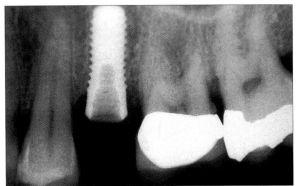

Fig 8   Radiograph immediately following implant placement.

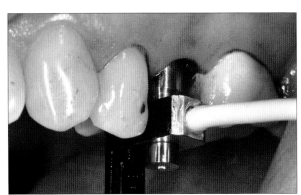

Fig 9   Resonance frequency analysis (RFA; Osstell mentor).

Subsequent to implant placement, a 4-mm solid abutment was positioned and torqued to 15 Ncm (Figs 10 – 11). Torquing was restricted to simplify the removal of the provisional restoration and the abutment subsequent to healing, in order to facilitate the making of a definitive synOcta impression of the osseointegrated implant. A provisional restoration was then fabricated and delivered. The provisional restoration was held short of contact with the opposing arch in maximum intercuspation and in all excursive movements (Figs 12 – 13).

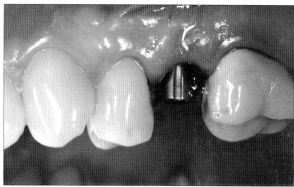

Fig 10 Placement of a 4-mm solid abutment (15 Ncm) to support the provisional restoration.

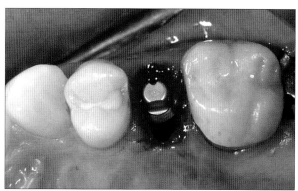

Fig 11 Occlusal view of the immediately placed implant and temporary abutment.

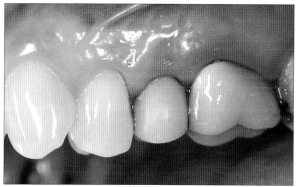

Fig 12 Lateral view of immediate restoration at the time of delivery.

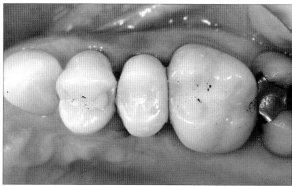

Fig 13 Occlusal view of immediate restoration at the time of delivery.

The patient was evaluated 8 weeks subsequent to the placement of the implant and provisional restoration. The soft tissues were considered to be in good health, and the implant was considered stable (Figs 14 – 16).

An implant-level (synOcta) impression was made in polyvinyl siloxane (Fig 17). A cast was poured in type IV dental stone and articulated using the appropriate dental records (Figs 18 – 19).

According to the ITI Consensus, implant restorations in the posterior regions of the mouth should be cemented where possible to improve their structural integrity and passivity. It is, however, also recommended that restorations be screw-retained if the implant shoulder is greater than 2 mm apical to the free gingival margin. This recommendation is given because it is not possible to remove residual cement at these depths. In this instance, the implant position was considered to be inappropriate for cementation to the depth of the shoulder on the proximal and palatal aspects. In order to maintain the advantages of improved passivity, occlusal surface form and strength, cementation of the definitive crown remained desirable.

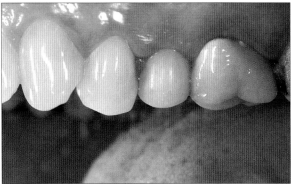

Fig 14 Lateral view 8 weeks subsequent to the placement of the implant.

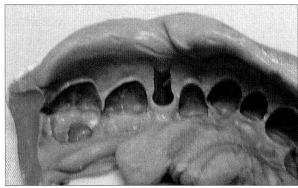

Fig 17 Implant-level (synOcta) impression of the implant in position 25.

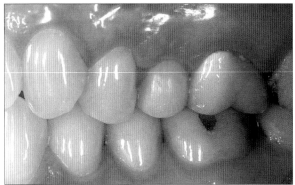

Fig 15 Lateral view (maximum intercuspation) 8 weeks subsequent to the placement of the implant.

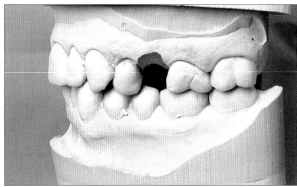

Fig 18 Lateral view of articulated casts.

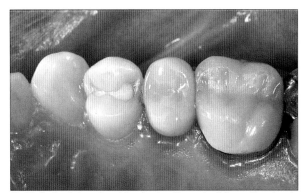

Fig 16 Occlusal view of provisional restoration and soft tissues 8 weeks subsequent to the placement of the implant.

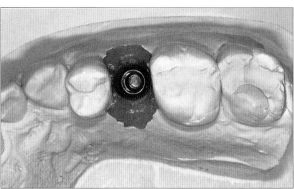

Fig 19 Occlusal view of articulated casts.

The incorporation of a customized titanium mesoabutment (Fig 20) allows for screw retention of the restoration at the shoulder level of the implant, and cementation of the final crown. The mesoabutment requires modification to provide a shaped restorative margin that is positioned slightly apical to the free gingival margin on the facial and proximal surfaces, and equigingival or slightly supragingival on the palatal aspect (Figs 21 – 23).

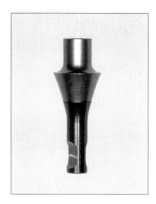

Fig 20 Titanium mesoabutment on the implant analog.

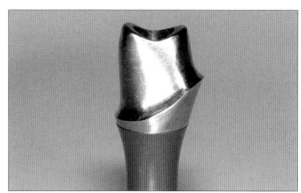

Fig 21 Modified mesoabutment. Note the scalloped form of the proposed crown margin.

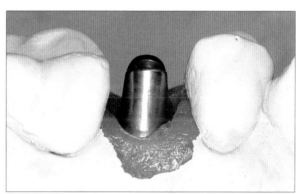

Fig 22 Facial aspect of customized mesoabutment displaying the subgingival position of the cement margin.

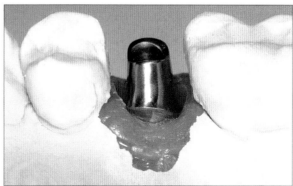

Fig 23 Palatal aspect of customized mesoabutment displaying the supragingival position of the cement margin.

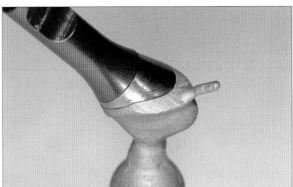

Fig 24 Cast framework adapted to the customized mesoabutment.

Following the final finishing of the customized mesoabut-ment, a metal-ceramic crown can be fabricated. Initially, a pattern for the framework is waxed up and cast in a high-noble alloy (Fig 24). The ceramic veneer is then fused to the framework according to the functional and esthet-ic demands of the restoration and the patient (Figs 25 – 26).

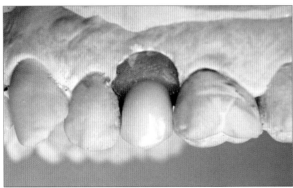

Fig 25 Lateral view of the finished metal-ceramic crown.

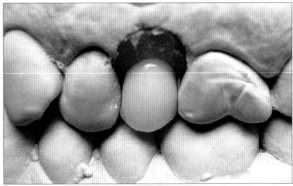

Fig 26 Lateral view of the finished metal-ceramic crown in maximum inter-cuspation.

Subsequent to the removal of the provisional restoration and the temporary solid abutment, the implant was irrigated with the air-water syringe and dried. The customized abutment was then positioned and, after the verification of the fit and esthetic outcome of the crown, torqued to 35 Ncm (Figs 27 – 28). The screw access hole was then obturated with a cotton pellet and sealed with a temporary restorative material. The definitive crown was then luted to place with a permanent cement (Fig 29). The occlusion was modified to ensure the drag of shimstock in maximum intercuspation and an absence of contacts in excursive movements. The implant and restoration remained functional and esthetically pleasing through four years of follow-up (Figs 30 – 31).

Acknowledgments

Laboratory Procedures
Todd A. Fridrich – Definitive Dental Arts, Coralville, Iowa, USA.

General Dental Procedures
Dr. Jack S. Jones – University of Florida, Gainesville, Florida, USA.

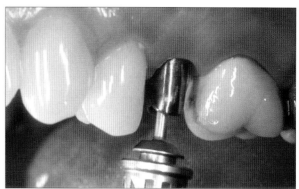

Fig 27 Placement and torquing of the customized mesoabutment.

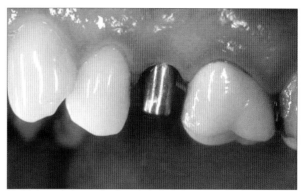

Fig 28 Lateral view confirming subgingival placement of facial margin.

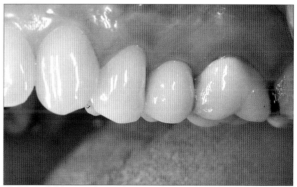

Fig 29 Definitive metal-ceramic restoration on the day of delivery.

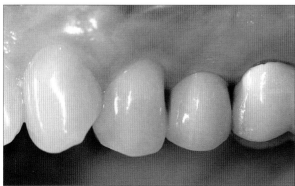

Fig 30 Definitive metal-ceramic restoration. Four-year follow-up.

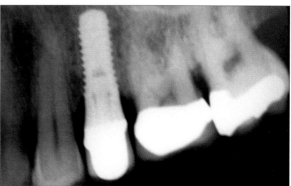

Fig 31 Radiographic at four-year follow-up.

4.8 Replacement of a Maxillary Right First Molar Using an Early Loading Protocol

B. Schmid

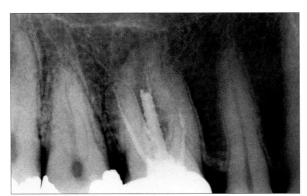

Fig 1   Periapical radiograph of tooth 16.

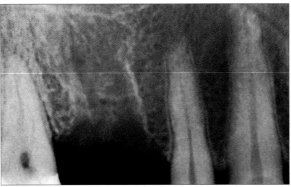

Fig 2   Implant site 2 months after the extraction of tooth 16.

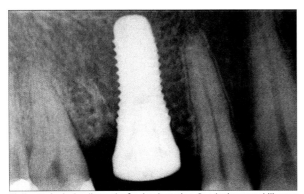

Fig 3   Periapical radiograph after implantation. Good primary stability was achieved at implant placement.

A 50-year-old female patient, a non-smoker, presented to the private office with a crown-restored and endodontically treated tooth, 16. Due to pain symptoms, there was a need for treatment. Another clinician had previously offered the patient a treatment option including root-canal retreatment and/or apical root resection, and she requested a second opinion.

Radiographic examination revealed a less than ideal root-canal therapy that had caused periapical osteolysis (Fig 1). After evaluating all the different treatment options, it was decided to extract tooth 16 and replace it with a dental implant and crown.

Two months after tooth extraction, a follow-up radiograph was taken to evaluate the bone fill in the extraction socket (Fig 2).

To avoid difficulties in implant positioning and anchoring due to premature, soft bone in the extraction site, a decision was made to postpone implant placement. This would provide the newly formed bone more time to mature.

Four months after tooth extraction, a Straumann Tapered Effect implant (endosteal diameter, 4.8 mm; length, 12 mm; Wide Neck prosthetic platform, 6.5 mm) was placed in the extraction socket in a transmucosal mode, following a type 3 implant placement protocol (Hämmerle and coworkers, 2004). Good primary stability was achieved at implant placement.

After implant placement, the implant was closed with a healing cap (Fig 3) and allowed to integrate non-submerged for 6 weeks.

The patient's esthetic expectations were low, and she expressed the wish to keep the treatment cost as low as possible. Therefore, a decision was made together with the patient to do without any provisional restoration.

Six weeks after implant placement, the soft tissues presented healthy (Figs 4–5), and no signs of inflammation and no bleeding upon probing could be detected.

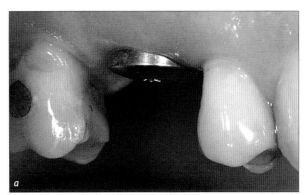

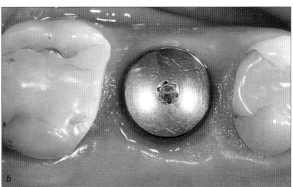

Figs 4a–b   Implantation site 6 weeks after implant placement before the removal of the healing cap for impression-making, lateral view, and occlusal view.

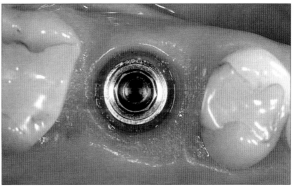

Fig 5   Soft-tissue status after the removal of the tissue former 6 weeks after placing the implant, occlusal view.

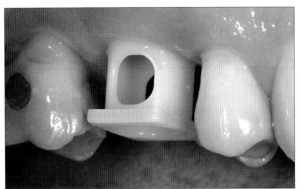

Fig 6a   Snap-on impression cap in place. The seating on the implant shoulder is considered correct if the impression cap can be smoothly spun on the implant shoulder.

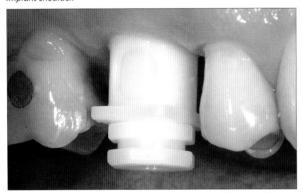

Fig 6b   The positioning cylinder is placed in the impression cap. The seating is considered correct when the positioning cylinder rests on the impression cap in a gap-free manner.

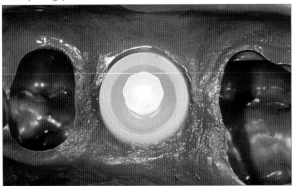

Fig 6c   The final impression before the pouring of the master cast.

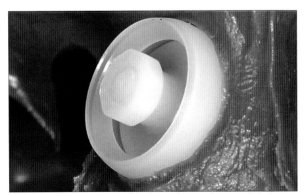

Fig 6d   Stable environment of the impression cap in terms of the impression material and the semi-submerged location of the implant shoulder.

All the clinical signs of a successfully integrated implant were present (Fig 5), so an impression was subsequently made for the fabrication of the final metal-ceramic crown (Fig 6). The loading of the implant 6 weeks after placement, follows an early-loading protocol (Ganeles and Wismeijer, 2004).

Due to the semi-submerged position of the implant and the resulting good accessibility of the implant shoulder, the snap-on impression technique was utilized.

In the dental laboratory, the analog was positioned on the impression cap (Fig 7) and the master cast was fabricated (Fig 8).

The coronal implant position allowed good access to the implant shoulder, thus a cement-retained crown, fabricated on a cementable synOcta abutment was possible (Figs 9 – 15).

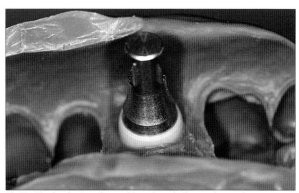

Fig 7   The implant analog positioned on the impression coping.

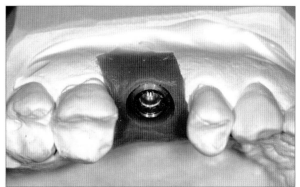

Fig 8   The implant analog in position 16 on the master cast.

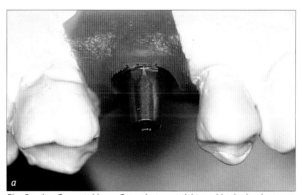

a

Figs 9a – b   Cementable synOcta abutment tightened in the implant analog.

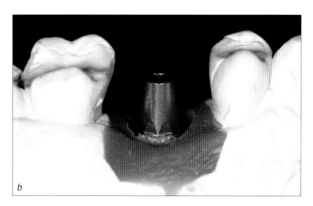

b

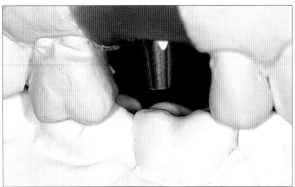

As there was sufficient interocclusal space, it was not necessary to shorten the abutment that was 5.5 mm high (Fig 10).

Fig 10 In full occlusion, the available space is favorable for crown fabrication.

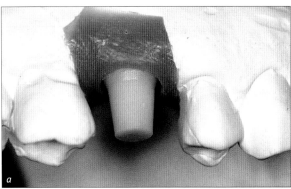
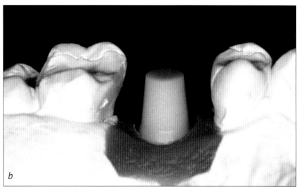

Figs 11a, b A plastic coping serves as the basis for the wax-up of the crown's metal core.

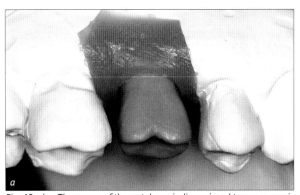
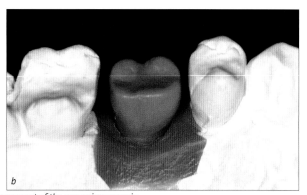

Figs 12a, b The wax-up of the metal core is dimensioned to ensure maximum support of the veneering ceramic.

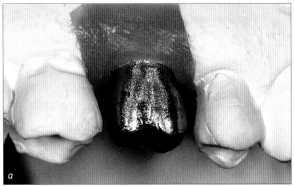
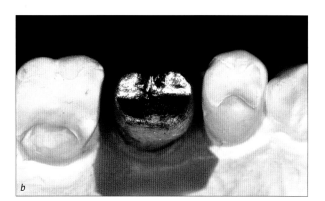

Figs 13a, b The metal core of the crown after trimming.

B. Schmid

In the laboratory, the occlusion was carefully checked and adjusted in order to ensure undisturbed static and dynamic occlusion (Fig 15).

After finalization, the crown and the abutment were delivered to the dentist. After the removal of the healing cap, the implant's internal octagon connection was cleaned with an alcohol-soaked piece of cotton wool and then thoroughly dried. Subsequently, the abutment was inserted into the implant and tightened to 35 Ncm (Fig 16).

Before the cementation of the final crown, the abutment's screw access channel was sealed with a small piece of cotton wool, followed by wax, to maintain access to the abutment screw.

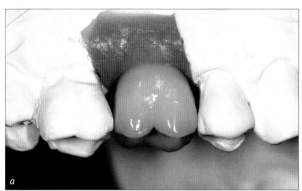
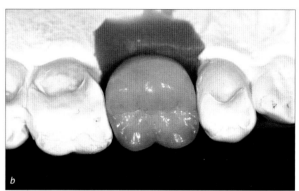

Figs 14a – b   The final metal-ceramic crown on the master cast. Care was taken to ensure adequate interproximal contacts for the passive seating of the crown.

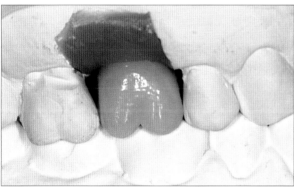

Fig 15   The final crown in full occlusal contact.

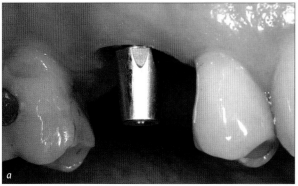
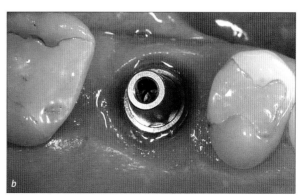

Figs 16a, b   The cementable synOcta abutment in situ, lateral view and occlusal view.

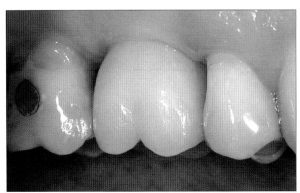

Fig 17   The crown blends into the row of natural teeth very nicely. Slight blanching of the buccal mucosa immediately after cementation is visible.

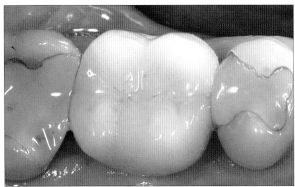

Fig 18   The final cement-retained metal-ceramic crown in situ. Occlusal view.

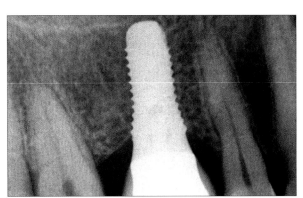

Fig 19   The final crown in situ. Precise seating on the implant shoulder is shown. Peri-implant bone crest levels are stable when compared to the post-implantation radiograph.

After the cementation of the final crown (Fig 17) and thorough removal of all cement remnants, the occlusion was carefully checked and final minor adjustments were made in the patient's mouth (Fig 18).

The periapical radiograph, taken after the cementation of the final crown, confirmed gap-free seating of the crown on the implant shoulder. No cement remnants were visible (Fig 19).

The 5-year follow-up photographs confirmed stable soft-tissue and bone conditions (Figs 20 – 21).

This particular clinical case allowed the application of a straightforward treatment protocol with regard to the surgical procedure as well as the prosthetic approach. Due to advanced socket healing at the time of surgery (4 months after tooth extraction), there was mature bone at the implantation site as well as almost completed bone remodeling. Therefore, the implant placement procedure was predictable with regard to implant positioning and the achievement of primary stability. Due to the transmucosal healing mode, the need for re-entry surgery was eliminated, thus reducing the number of surgical interventions to one. Furthermore, the posterior location of the implantation site and the patient's low esthetic expectations allowed for a healing period without provisional restoration, since soft tissue conditioning by means of a provisional crown was not an objective.

The implant shoulder was easy to access thanks to its transmucosal position. This allowed for the application of the snap-on impression technique as well as the insertion of a cement-retained crown on a prefabricated, non-individualized abutment.

In summary, the main advantages of the chosen treatment protocol are: the reduction of treatment steps, low overall treatment cost, and a relatively short treatment period. The surgical and the restorative procedures pursued in this case can be classified as straightforward due to the low difficulty and risk associated with the treatment.

Acknowledgments

Laboratory Procedures
Beat Heckendorn – Master Dental Technician, Bern, Switzerland.

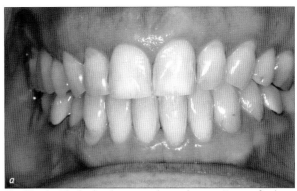

Figs 20a – b   The implant-borne metal ceramic crown 5 years after insertion, full-mouth view and occlusal aspect.

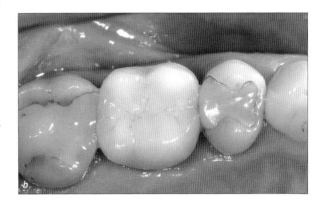

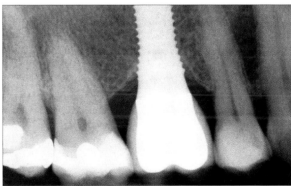

Fig 21   5 years after implant placement, the periapical radiograph documents stable peri-implant bone levels.

4.9 Replacement of a Maxillary Right Second Premolar Using an Early Loading Protocol

M. Roccuzzo

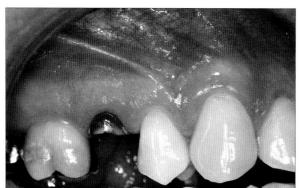

Fig 1   The initial clinical situation after the tooth fracture.

In February 2002, a 31-year-old non-smoking male patient was referred by his dentist after the fracture of the crown of the maxillary right second premolar, tooth 15 (Fig 1).

The fracture line was located apically to the gingival margin, particularly on the palatal side (Fig 2).

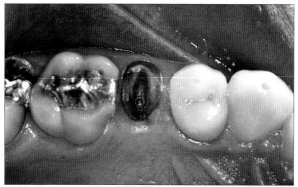

Fig 2   The poor condition of the endodontically treated root in combination with the unfavorable, mostly subgingival course of the fracture line would aggravate prosthetic restoration without adjunctive treatment such as orthodontic root extrusion.

Radiographic examination revealed the presence of a previous endodontic treatment with a non-ideal apical seal. There were no signs of periapical osteolysis. The level of the interproximal bone was normal (Fig 3).

The patient's medical history did not reveal any significant findings and he was in good general health. Different therapeutic options were discussed with the patient:

- Option 1: Traditional prosthetic reconstruction with a three-unit fixed dental prosthesis.
- Option 2: The orthodontic extrusion of the root to extend the clinical crown.
- Option 3: The extraction of the root and subsequent implant placement in combination with an appropriate loading protocol.

The patient, who worked as a TV cameraman with a significant travel schedule, expressed the desire to keep the number of surgical procedures to a minimum and to limit the time with no tooth. A thorough examination of the site revealed healthy, edema-free gingiva and the absence of periodontal pockets on the teeth adjacent to the fractured tooth. The patient was therefore informed about the possibility of inserting a Straumann Tapered Effect (TE) implant into the extraction socket immediately after the removal of the root (type 1 implant placement protocol (Hämmerle and coworkers, 2004)). Subsequently, the patient gave his informed consent for this treatment.

After administration of local anesthesia, a full-thickness flap was elevated on the palatal aspect of the alveolar ridge to expose the alveolar bone. Sutures were used for flap retraction. The incision was carried out on the palatal aspect of the ridge and limited to three teeth. On the facial aspect, no incision was made in order to reduce the risk of buccal soft tissue recession. The root was extracted with a minimally invasive mode to preserve the surrounding tissues, particularly the buccal bone. The mesiodistal and the vestibulopalatal dimensions of the alveolus were measured (Fig 4) and they allowed for the immediate placement of a Straumann Tapered Effect implant (endosteal diameter, 4.1 mm; length, 12 mm; Regular Neck prosthetic platform, 4.8 mm).

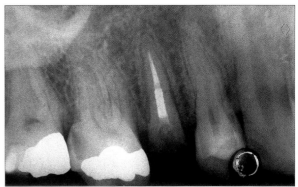

Fig 3 Periapical radiograph of tooth 15 prior to the minimally traumatic removal of the root remnant.

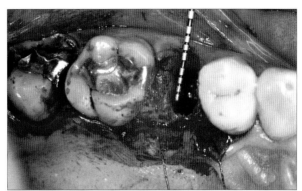

Fig 4 Situation after the minimally traumatic extraction of the root. The alveolar walls are intact. The soft tissues on the facial aspect of the extraction site were not touched.

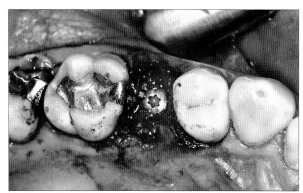
Fig 5 Situation after the application of bone substitute material.

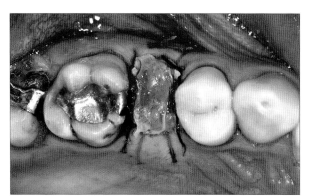
Fig 6 The implant site after coverage and careful suturing.

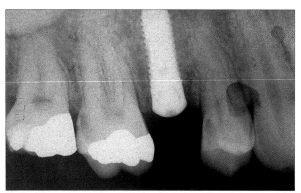
Fig 7 The post-surgical periapical radiograph confirmed the correct implant position.

Initial rotary site preparation was minimized to facilitate the use of osteotomes in the sites. Screw taps were not used. The implant was manually inserted in a self-tapping fashion, and primary stability was achieved. The implant was placed with the border of the SLA surface slightly apical to the alveolar bone crest, positioning the machined neck portion in a transmucosal manner. A closure screw was inserted into the implant. The space between the implant and the alveolar walls was filled with deproteinized bovine bone granules (Bio-Oss, Geistlich), and the flap was sutured with no intention to submerge the implant, carefully adapting the soft tissues to support the augmentation material (Fig 5). Based on the type 1 implant placement protocol, the complexity of this case is considered advanced.

Subsequently, the site was covered with a few drops of a flowable polylactide polymer (Atrisorb, Atrix Laboratories). After application, the material barrier was misted with a fine spray of sterile saline solution for solidification, to function as a barrier and prevent the dislocation of the bone substitute (Fig 6).

The radiographic examination, performed immediately after surgery, confirmed the correct positioning of the implant (Fig 7).

The patient was advised to discontinue tooth brushing and to avoid trauma in the site of surgery for the first 3 weeks. He was also instructed to rinse with 0.2% chlorhexidine digluconate solution for 1 minute three times a day for the same period of time. The protection and sutures were removed 10 days after surgery.

Three weeks after the implant placement, the patient was instructed to start thoroughly brushing his teeth in order to ensure adequate plaque control to minimize the risk for soft tissue recession and the exposure of the coronal parts of the implant's neck portion.

Six weeks after surgery, the peri-implant mucosa appeared healthy and free from inflammation. Probing depth was within the physiological limit around both the implant and the adjacent teeth. Plaque control was adequate, and there was no bleeding on probing (Figs 8a,b).

At the same time, a solid abutment was inserted into the implant and tightened to 35 Ncm in order to proceed with the provisional restoration. The impression was made with a snap-on impression cap and a positioning cylinder to transfer the oral position of the implant to the master cast (Figs 9 – 13).

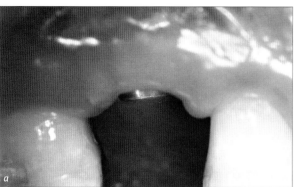

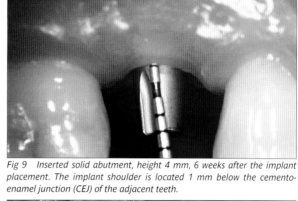

Figs 8a – b   At 6 weeks after the implant placement, the peri-implant soft tissues were healthy and stable. The implantation site had healed uneventfully.

Fig 9   Inserted solid abutment, height 4 mm, 6 weeks after the implant placement. The implant shoulder is located 1 mm below the cemento-enamel junction (CEJ) of the adjacent teeth.

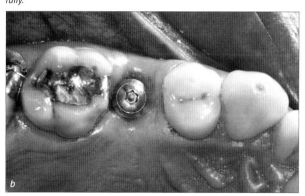

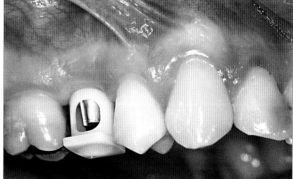

Fig 10   The impression cap is placed on the implant shoulder. Precise seating is confirmed by carefully turning the cap on the implant. If this is possible in a smooth, non-interrupted way, the impression cap sits on the implant shoulder precisely.

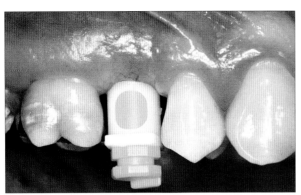

Fig 11   The yellow positioning cylinder is positioned on top of the solid abutment. Care is taken to ensure gap-free seating on the coronal portion of the impression cap.

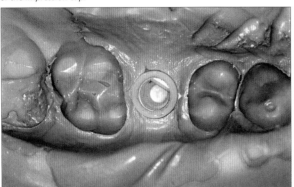

Fig 12   The impression, ready for the pouring of the master cast.

The provisional crown was cemented on the solid abutment according to an early loading protocol (Roccuzzo and coworkers, 2001). Provisionals should be kept in place for at least a month in order to facilitate soft tissue maturation for an ideal final esthetic restoration. The convexity of the provisional's buccal profile determines the height of the mucosal margin (Fig 14).

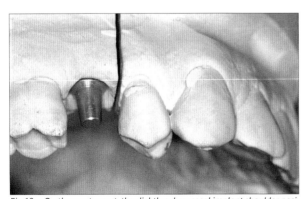

Fig 13   On the master cast, the slightly submucosal implant shoulder position is visible, allowing for a submucosal crown margin position. The implant shoulder region is accessible for later cement removal.

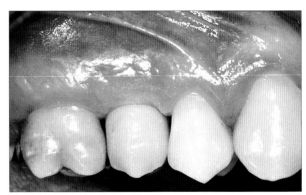

Fig 14   The provisional crown remained in situ for 8 weeks in order to allow for sufficient soft-tissue maturation. At this point of the treatment, the shape of the provisional crown follows functional rather than esthetic aspects in order to facilitate esthetic soft-tissue maturation.

Two months after the cementation of the provisional crown, a metal-ceramic crown was completed and cemented (Figs 15–16).

After the cementation of the final crown, cement remnants were thoroughly removed. Gap-free seating of the final crown on the implant shoulder was confirmed on the post-cementation periapical radiograph (Fig 16).

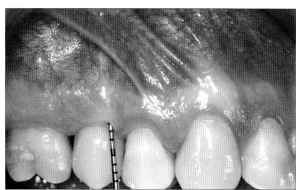

Fig 15   The final metal ceramic crown in situ 2 months after the implant placement. The peri-implant soft tissues are healthy.

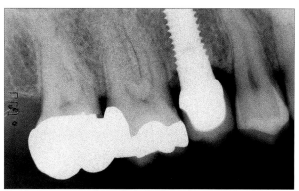

Fig 16   Post-cementation periapical radiograph. At 2 months after the implant placement, the implant is well integrated. Peri-implant bone structures are stable.

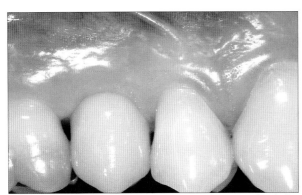

Fig 17   Clinical situation at the follow-up examination 1 year after the implant placement.

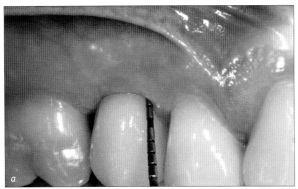

Figs 18a–b   Clinical situation and periapical radiograph at the follow-up examination 3 years after the implant placement.

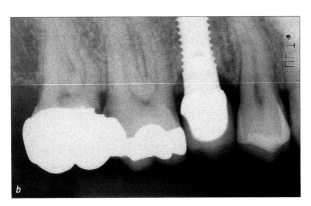

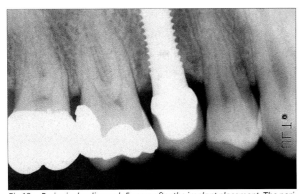

Fig 19   Periapical radiograph 5 years after the implant placement. The peri-implant bone levels are stable.

The patient was recalled at various intervals for clinical examination. At these opportunities, professional cleansing was performed as necessary. Clinical and radiographic examinations were carried out at 1, 3, and 5 years (Figs 17–20).

The following benefits could be provided to the patient with the treatment protocol – immediate implant placement and early-loading protocol – chosen in this case:

- Reduction of the surgical interventions to the absolute minimum of 1 by choosing an immediate placement protocol in combination with a non-submerged healing mode.
- Shortening of the toothless phase due to an early loading protocol with implant loading 7 weeks after implant placement.
- Reduction of the overall treatment cost by abstaining from the fabrication of a removable partial denture to close the gap in position 15.

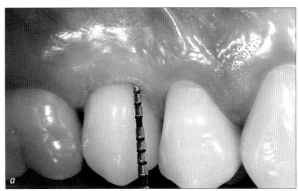

Figs 20a – b   Clinical appearance of the implant site 5 years after implant placement. The peri-implant mucosa is healthy and stable.

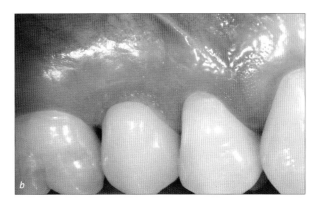

Acknowledgments
The help of Dr. Marco Bunino, Dr. Paolo Lo Giudice, and Lab Technician Gianpiero Sorgarello is greatly appreciated.

4.10 Replacement of a Maxillary Left First Molar Using an Early Loading Protocol

D. Buser, C. Hart

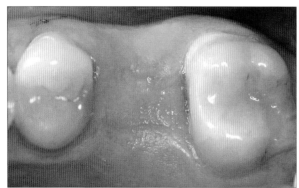

Fig 1   Missing maxillary first molar at position 26.

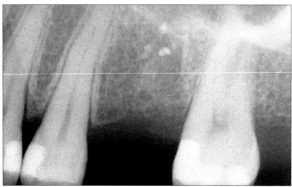

Fig 2   Preoperative radiograph six months following extraction.

A 28-year-old female patient was referred to our clinic for replacement of the upper left first molar with a dental implant and crown (Fig 1). The tooth had been removed six months before because of an endodontic complication. The patient's main requests were restoration of her masticatory function and closure of the tooth gap at position 26.

The patient was in good general health, and her medical history was without significant findings. There were no obstacles to implant therapy. The preoperative radiograph revealed a bone height sufficient for implant placement in a largely healed extraction socket with some endodontic filling material residue (Fig 2).

The mesiodistal gap size and the bone height and crest width at position 26 permitted the placement of a Straumann Standard Wide Neck implant (endosteal diameter, 4.8 mm; length, 10 mm; WN prosthetic platform, 6.5 mm). The decision was made to use the Straumann SLActive implant surface, which is characterized by rapid bone integration. Given sufficient implant stability, early implant loading – as soon as three weeks after placement – can be considered.

Figure 3 shows the clinical situation immediately after implant placement. Good primary implant stability was achieved during placement, as verified with the Osstell mentor device (Integration Diagnostics AB, Göteborg), which confirmed excellent primary stability with an implant stability quotient (ISQ) of 70 (Figs 4–5).

The implant was placed in a coronoapical position that allowed for non-submerged healing. Before the adaptation of the wound margins, a Wide Neck healing cap was inserted (Fig 6). To ensure a precise, tension-free adaptation of the wound margins around the implant's neck portion, two small pedicle flaps were prepared and adapted around the implant neck (Fig 6).

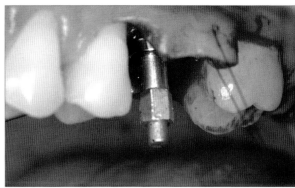

Fig 4   The magnetic, metallic Smartpeg post was inserted to measure the ISQ.

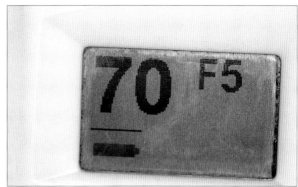

Fig 5   The ISQ on the Osstell mentor display.

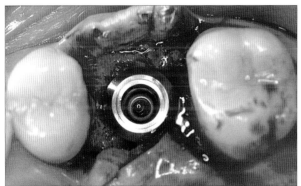

Fig 3   The implant at site 26 immediately after placement. The mesiodistal gap width of > 8.5 mm in combination with the orofacial crestal width of > 6.8 mm and sufficient vertical bone height permitted the placement of a Wide Neck implant with a length of 10 mm.

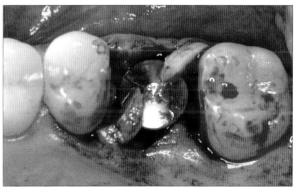

Fig 6   The preparation of two pedicle flaps allows for a precise, tension-free wound-margin adaptation around the implant neck.

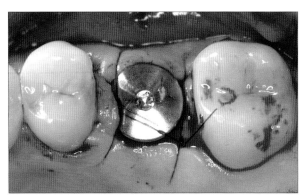

Fig 7   The implant site after soft tissue suturing.

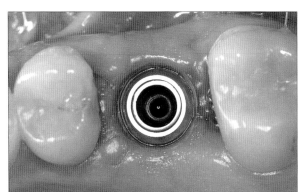

Fig 8   Clinical status three weeks after implant placement.

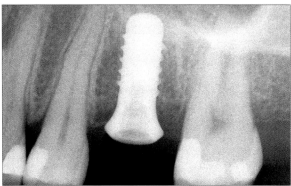

Fig 9   The corresponding radiograph of day 21 demonstrating normal bone integration.

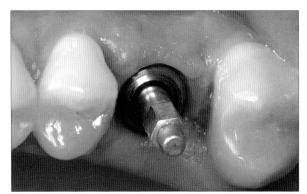

Fig 10   Clinical situation following the insertion of a Smartpeg post for measuring the ISQ.

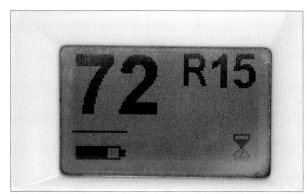

Fig 11   An ISQ of 72 on day 21 permits loading the restoration with a crown within one week.

Subsequently, the peri-implant soft tissues were stabilized with two interrupted 5.0 sutures (Fig 7).

The sutures were removed on day 7, and the patient received instructions for home-care procedures for the implant site. Three weeks after placement, the healing of the peri-implant soft tissues had progressed nicely (Fig 8).

The periapical radiograph showed normal bone integration of the implant (Fig 9). Ankylotic stability was confirmed by a light tapping sound.

At this time, implant stability was checked again with the Osstell mentor device (Fig 10).

The ISQ of 72 (Fig 11) confirmed good bone integration of the Wide Neck implant and permitted an impression to be made on day 21. It was decided to fabricate the definitive crown as planned.

An impression was made subsequent to the implant stability measurement for the fabrication of a cemented ceramo-metal crown.

One week later, i.e. 4 weeks after the implant was placed, a Wide Neck cementable synOcta abutment was inserted and tightened to 35 Ncm (Fig 12). Due to the somewhat limited interocclusal space, the abutment, which was originally 5.5 mm in height, had to be slightly shortened by the dental technician.

During the same appointment, the metal-ceramic crown was cemented (Fig 13), thus applying an early loading protocol four weeks after implant placement. Care was taken to thoroughly remove any cement residue around the implant shoulder in order to avoid possible inflammatory reactions.

The periapical radiograph, taken immediately after the cementation of the crown, showed a well-integrated implant and precise, gap-free seating of the crown on the implant shoulder (Fig 14). The cement residue visible at the disto-cervical aspect of the crown was carefully removed.

Six months after implant placement, i.e. 5 months after implant loading, the peri-implant soft tissues had well adapted to the implant-supported crown (Fig 15). The peri-implant mucosa was firm and healthy, with no bleeding on probing.

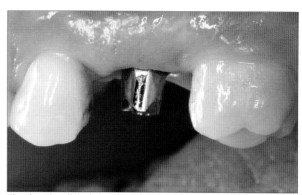

Fig 12   The clinical situation after the insertion of the Wide Neck cementable synOcta abutment for anchorage of a cemented metal-ceramic crown, 28 days after implant placement.

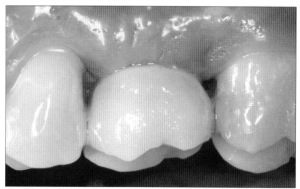

Fig 13   The lateral mirror view shows the implant crown immediately after seating. The peri-implant papillae will form within a few weeks.

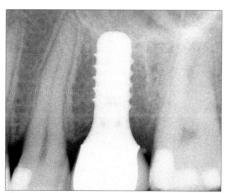

Fig 14   Periapical radiograph taken after the cementation of the final crown, 28 days after implant placement.

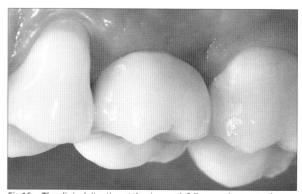

Fig 15   The clinical situation at the six-month follow-up, demonstrating stable and healthy peri-implant mucosa.

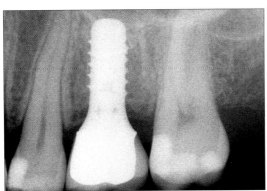

Fig 16   Periapical radiograph six months after implant placement.

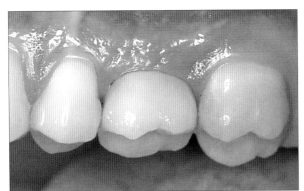

Fig 17   Clinical status at the one-year follow-up control, demonstrating healthy peri-implant soft tissues.

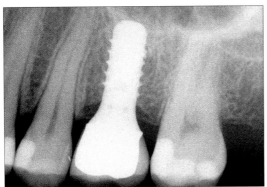

Fig 18   The corresponding radiograph at the one-year follow-up.

The periapical follow-up radiograph six months after implant placement confirmed a well-integrated implant with normal peri-implant bone structures and bone height (Fig 16).

The follow-up control at 12 months demonstrated healthy and stable peri-implant soft tissues at the implant crown (Fig 17).

The successful clinical status was confirmed by a periapical radiograph with a well-integrated implant and stable peri-implant bone crest levels (Fig 18).

The treatment and loading protocol described above provided the following advantages to the patient:

The surgical phase could be limited to one surgical intervention because of the non-submerged approach that permitted access to the implant shoulder without a re-opening procedure. Due to the location of the tooth gap and the otherwise full and functioning dentition, the patient's chewing function was only slightly compromised. Therefore, it was not necessary to provide the patient with a removable provisional denture for the healing periods after extraction and implant placement.

The Straumann SLActive implant surface accelerated osseointegration, so that an ISQ of 72 was reached three weeks after implant placement, which permitted an early loading protocol. Within a week, the final metal-ceramic crown was fabricated by the dental technician and incorporated with a cementable synOcta abutment. Hence, the overall healing period following implant placement was reduced to just four weeks without sacrificing the predictability and therefore the safety of the treatment. This approach was also attractive to the patient from an economic point of view, since this treatment offered an excellent cost/benefit ratio.

The surgical and the restorative procedures chosen for this patient can be categorized as straightforward (Cat. S) due to the relatively low difficulty and risk associated with this treatment.

Acknowledgments

Laboratory procedures
René Schaetzle – Master Dental Technician, Interlaken, Switzerland

Single-Tooth Gaps in the Anterior Maxilla

4.11 Replacement of a Maxillary Right Central Incisor Using an Immediate Restoration Protocol

C. Evans, A. Rosenberg

A healthy 54-year-old male was referred to a specialist prosthodontic clinic for the management of the maxillary right central incisor, tooth 11. It had been endodontically treated approximately 20 years before and was decoronated during trauma to the mouth (Fig 1). Emergency treatment provided by the referring general dentist provisionally restored the tooth with a prefabricated post and full coronal resin restoration.

The patient requested a fixed replacement of tooth 11. The patient displayed a moderate lip line and, on wide smiling, a display of the interproximal papilla, and 1 mm of cervical gingival margin.

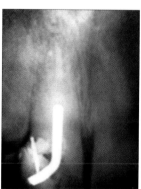

Fig 1   Periapical view of tooth 11 prior to trauma.

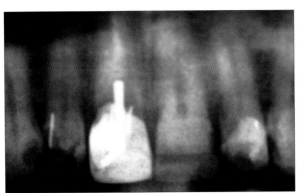

Fig 2   Orthopantomograph showing tooth 11 to be unrestorable.

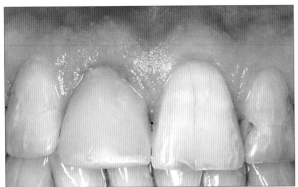

Fig 3   Tooth 11 restored with a resin crown after trauma.

Clinical examination revealed tooth 11 to be reconstructed with a resin crown with buccal and lingual restorative margins located 1 – 3 mm subgingivally (Fig 3). The tissue biotype was thick in nature and the cervical gingival margin was positioned about 0.5 – 1.0 mm further coronally than that of tooth 21. The adjacent teeth were restored with routine resin restorations. Radiographic examination showed a heavily filled central incisor with a short post and small periapical radiolucency (Fig 2).

A tapered coronal pulp chamber extended subcrestally into the pulp canal system. The tooth was deemed to be not restorable via conventional means and the options presented to the patient were a three-unit conventional fixed dental prosthesis or an implant-retained restoration. The patient's preference was to replace tooth 11 with an implant-retained restoration, and he requested a treatment approach that avoided the use of a removable interim restoration due to occupational commitments. Following careful clinical and radiographic assessment, tooth extraction in combination with immediate implant placement and provisional restoration was offered as a viable treatment option to the patient.

Due to the small size of the periapical lesion, the presence of good buccolingual and vertical bone available above the root apex, a favorable anterior occlusal relationship, and a cervical gingival margin more coronal than the contralateral tooth, the immediate protocol was assessed to present minimal risk to achieving an esthetic and functional outcome. In order for this treatment approach to be followed, the implant insertion torque was required to be greater than 35 Ncm to ensure excellent primary implant stability. The immediate provisional restoration was also planned to be free from direct occlusal contacts and the patient was required to follow a soft diet for 4 weeks after implant placement (Ganeles and Wismeijer, 2004). The patient was advised that if these requirements could not be met at the time of surgery, an immediate-restoration protocol would not be followed and a removable interim prosthesis would be required. Additionally, the risk of complications, such as wound infection, an increased risk of implant failure compared to delayed loading protocols, significant soft tissue recession, and provisional denture fracture and loosening, were discussed with the patient in detail (Berglundh and coworkers, 2002). These risks were acceptable to the patient.

The proposed treatment plan was to extract the crown and the root fragment of tooth 11 and to place a Straumann implant using an immediate placement/immediate restoration protocol. A provisional acrylic-resin implant-supported crown would be fabricated to restore the site immediately following implant placement. A definitive metal-ceramic crown would be fabricated after implant integration and the soft-tissue healing period of 6 months. The level of difficulty of the proposed treatment is considered "complex", as defined by the SAC classification (Buser and coworkers, 2004). Implant surgery in such cases is complex and requires that the surgeon ensures that the implant shoulder does not move buccally at any stage during implant insertion (Quirynen and coworkers, 2007). If this occurs, the final esthetic outcome will be compromised.

Prior to implant surgery, articulated study casts and shade selection for the provisional crown were made. A Regular Neck (RN) synOcta impression cap and an RN synOcta titanium post for temporary restorations were ordered and received.

Minimally traumatic crown and root removal using fine osteotomes and a flapless approach was performed under local anesthesia. The extraction site was carefully examined visually and with a periodontal probe to ensure that the buccal plate of bone was intact and not perforated. Osteotomy preparation was performed under copious irrigation to allow the placement of the implant shoulder 2 – 3 mm apical to the planned cervical crown margin and with an axial inclination to facilitate lingual screw access for the final restoration. The extraction site was prepared with the drill angled into the palatal wall of the extraction socket to prevent the existing socket anatomy dictating the final implant position. The coronal aspect of the palatal wall was countersunk to prevent the tulip-shaped implant collar flaring the implant buccally during the final stages of implant insertion. A Straumann Standard Plus implant (endosteal diameter, 4.1 mm; length, 12 mm; Regular Neck prosthetic platform, 4.8 mm) with SLA surface was placed with a final insertion torque greater than 35 Ncm. An RN synOcta impression cap was milled to reduce the diameter of the impression coping at the implant shoulder, taking care not to damage the shoulder fit surface. This reduces the potential of the coping binding to the crestal bone and it allows the coping to seat fully. The impression cap was then attached to the implant and a transfer pick-up made using silicone bite-registration material (Figs 4 – 6).

A 3-mm RN healing cap was attached to the implant using a light hand torque (Fig 7).

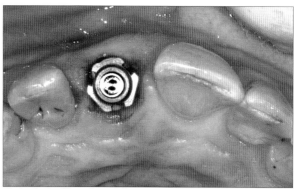
Fig 4   Optimal buccolingual placement.

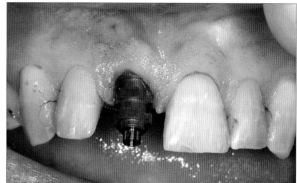
Fig 5   The inserted impression cap.

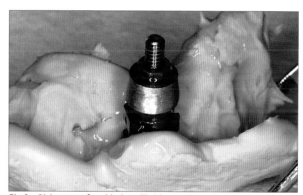
Fig 6   Pickup transfer with the milled impression cap.

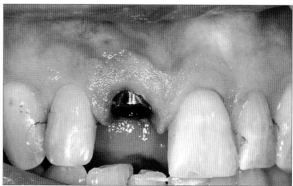
Fig 7   The healing cap, hand-tightened.

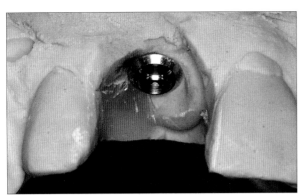

Fig 8   Laboratory analog.

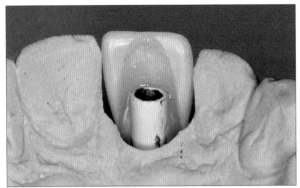

Fig 9   The acrylic denture tooth was trimmed and grit-blasted; the temporary coping was opaqued and ready to process.

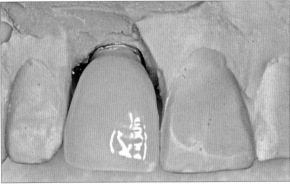

Fig 10   The completed provisional.

In the dental laboratory, a RN synOcta laboratory analog was connected to the impression cap and the master cast modified through the removal of tooth 11. The base below the tooth was also cut away to allow a passive fit of the impression cap with the analog attached without stone impingement. Fast-setting stone was then poured around the cap to form a working cast (Fig 8).

The titanium RN synOcta post for temporary restorations was modified and opaqued. An acrylic-resin denture tooth (Vitapan Lumin Acryl) was trimmed to fit and processed with acrylic resin (Palapress, Heraeus Kulzer) over the cap to form a screw-retained provisional crown (Figs 9 – 10).

The submergence profile was then adjusted (Fig 11) and the crown delivered to the patient using the torque control device and SCS screwdriver to apply a force of 20 Ncm (Fig 12). The occlusion was adjusted to avoid direct contact in protrusive movement. Post-insertion instructions were provided to the patient to avoid eating firm food and to avoid buccally directed leverage forces being applied to the crown. The patient was followed 1 week, 1 month, and 3 months (Fig 13) after temporary restoration. Radiographs were taken at 1 month and 3 months.

The definitive restoration of the implant commenced 6 months after extraction, when the peri-implant tissue contours were stable (Fig 14). An implant level impression was made using an RN synOcta impression cap with GC pattern resin applied to the gingival portion to capture the gingival profile developed by the temporary crown (Fig 15).

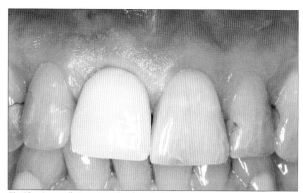

Fig 12   Immediate restoration inserted.

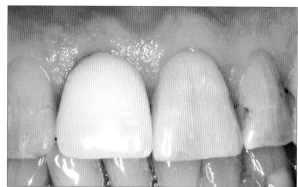

Fig 13   The provisional restoration 3 months after insertion.

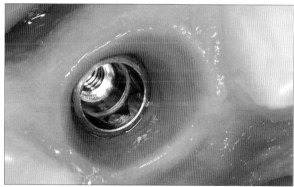

Fig 14   Soft-tissue contouring from the provisional.

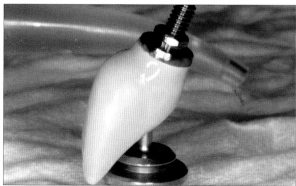

Fig 11   The submergence profile adjusted to reduce tissue blanching.

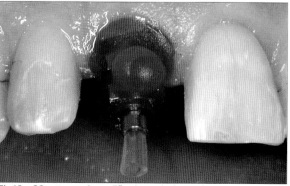

Fig 15   GC pattern resin modification to the impression cap to augment retention in the impression and capture the soft-tissue profile.

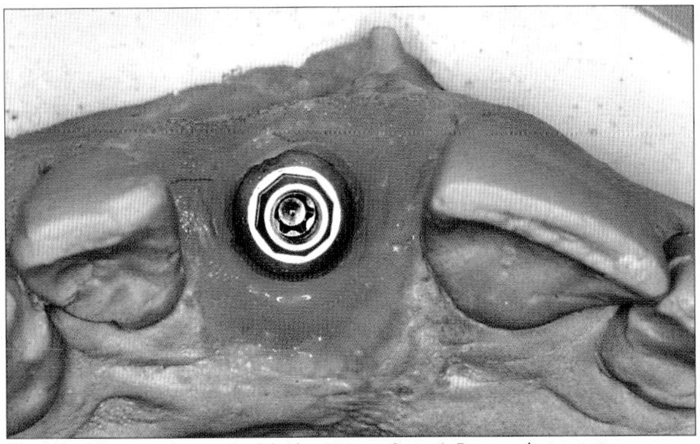

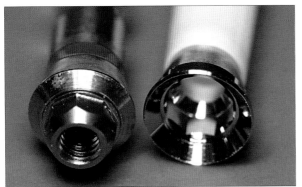

Fig 16   The master cast with the RN synOcta 1.5-mm abutment.

The RN synOcta laboratory analog was connected to the impression cap in the final impression and the master cast poured in type 4 dental stone (Prima Rock, Whip Mix). After the model articulation, the decision was made to proceed with a palatal screw-retained metal-ceramic crown, as planned during the case assessment. An RN synOcta 1.5-mm abutment was selected (Fig 16) and an RN synOcta gold coping for crowns was connected and waxed to provide the metal framework design suitable for a metal-ceramic crown (Fig 17). Using a lost wax casting technique, precious bonding alloy (PontoLloyd P, Bego) was cast to the gold coping (Fig 18). Ceramic material was built over the framework (Vita VM13) to develop a metal-ceramic screw-retained crown with a submergence profile similar to that of the provisional crown (Fig 19).

At the insertion appointment, the provisional implant-supported denture was removed and the RN synOcta 1.5-mm abutment was tightened to 35 Ncm. The final crown was adjusted for proximal and occlusal contacts and delivered with the occlusal screw tightened to 15 Ncm. A follow-up periapical radiograph taken after 18 months demonstrates stable peri-implant bone levels (Fig 20).

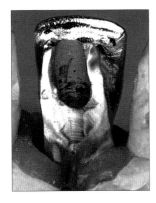

Fig 17   RN synOcta analog with the 1.5 mm synOcta abutment connected and an RN synOcta gold coping for crowns.

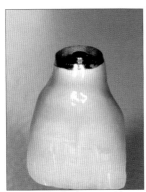

Fig 18   The RN synOcta gold coping casting.

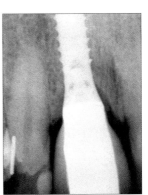

Fig 19   The final crown with contours similar to the provisional.

Fig 20   Stable peri-implant bone levels at 18 months.

A pleasing esthetic result was achieved through ideal implant placement and careful soft-tissue manipulation during the final stages of temporization (Fig 21). The soft tissue result is stable at 18 months (Fig 22). A follow-up periapical radiograph taken after 24 months confirms stable periimplant bone levels (Fig 23).

The immediate treatment protocol followed for this case provided the patient a cost-effective treatment outcome that obviated the need for a removable interim restoration. This reduced the overall treatment cost to the patient as well as the treatment time.

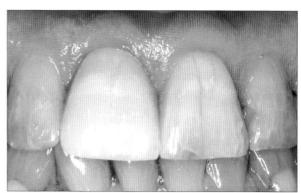

Fig 21   The final restoration after 18 months in function.

Acknowledgments

Laboratory Procedures
Mark Davis and James Brown – Asling Laboratory, Melbourne, Australia.

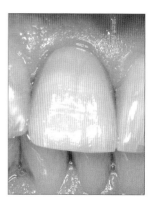

Fig 22   Stable peri-implant tissues at 18 months.

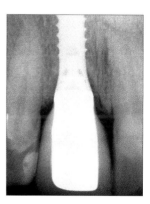

Fig 23   Radiograph at 24 months.

4.12 Replacement of a Maxillary Right Central Incisor Using an Early Loading Protocol

D. Morton, J. Ruskin

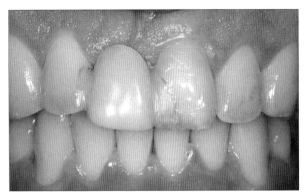

Fig 1   Pre-treatment retracted anterior view.

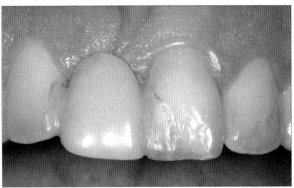

Fig 2   Pre-treatment retracted view, maxillary anterior segment.

This 23-year-old male presented for consultation and treatment for a missing maxillary right central incisor (tooth 11). His medical history was significant for asthma and light cigarette smoking (a quarter of a pack per day for three to five years). The patient had previously received orthodontic therapy to improve tooth alignment and was satisfied with the esthetic outcome.

His periodontal status was considered to be excellent, and his tissue biotype was considered to be thick (Figs 1 – 2). His esthetic demands were reasonable and he expressed the desire for a more permanent tooth replacement. The maxillary right central incisor had been lost due to trauma at approximately age 10, and had been originally replaced with a composite-resin interim prosthesis retained by the left central incisor. This had fractured and been replaced by an acrylic resin tooth bonded directly to the retainer (Figs 1 – 2). His maxillary anterior segment was characterized by gingival disharmony, mostly associated with the right lateral incisor. The patient did not wish to pursue additional orthodontic therapy to improve tooth alignment and gingival symmetry.

The patient was given several treatment options. These included:

- Option 1: A definitive metal-ceramic, cantilevered fixed dental prosthesis retained by the left central incisor.
- Option 2: A definitive metal-ceramic resin-retained fixed dental prosthesis.
- Option 3: An implant-supported and retained crown, replacing tooth 11, accompanied by a single crown on tooth 21.

The patient elected and consented to pursue the implant-supported and retained treatment option, in addition to a crown on the adjacent tooth. The existing prosthesis was therefore removed, and the left central incisor evaluated and considered to be healthy and capable of supporting a full-coverage restoration (Fig 3). Irreversible hydrocolloid impressions were obtained and poured in low expansion dental stone, and a provisional fixed dental prosthesis was fabricated and delivered (Fig 4).

The casts were utilized for the fabrication of a surgical template, which was used to communicate the desired position of the implant in the orofacial and mesiodestal dimensions (Fig 5). The provisional restoration was utilized to communicate the desired implant-shoulder depth (Fig 6).

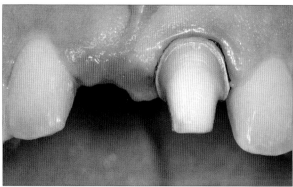

Fig 3   Anterior view of site 11 and the adjacent tooth.

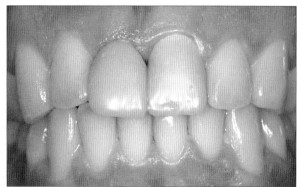

Fig 4   Provisional fixed dental prosthesis at the four-week follow-up.

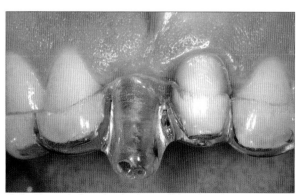

Fig 5   The surgical template in place, verifying adaptation.

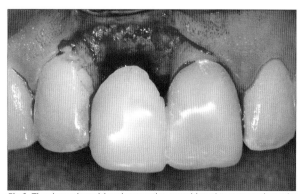

Fig 6 The cleaned provisional restoration repositioned to communicate the desired implant shoulder depth (2 mm apical to planned gingival margin).

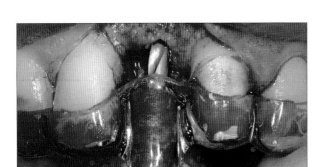

Fig 7   Preparation of the implant bed utilizing the surgical template.

A Straumann Standard Plus implant (endosteal diameter, 4.1 mm; length, 10 mm; Regular Neck prosthetic platform, 4.8 mm) was positioned according to the template, with an implant shoulder depth approximately 2 mm apical to the margin of the provisional restoration and 1 mm apical to the planned margin of the adjacent restoration (Figs 7–8). A closure screw was inserted, the wound was closed, and the provisional restoration was replaced (Fig 9). A radiograph was then obtained, confirming the appropriate position of the implant (Fig 10).

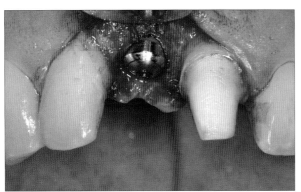

Fig 8   The implant in position.

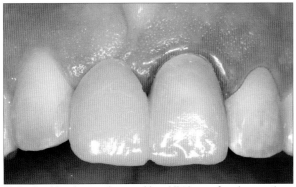

Fig 9   Provisional restoration repositioned (24 hours after placement).

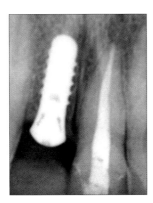

Fig 10   Radiograph after implant placement.

The implant was allowed to heal undisturbed for 6 weeks. The provisional restoration was then carefully removed and the site evaluated (Fig 11). The soft tissue health was considered appropriate for the surgical exposure of the implant, and the creation of the emergence profile with an implant-supported provisional prosthesis. Prior to the surgical exposure of the implant, photographs were made of the adjacent teeth to record surface characteristics, and with a tab to record the selected shade (Figs 12 – 13).

A 5-mm tissue punch was used to gain access to the implant. Care was taken to ensure that the punch was positioned appropriately towards the palatal aspect of the region above the implant in order to prevent irreversible loss of facial soft tissue. In addition, the punch was positioned equidistant from the adjacent teeth to prevent impingement upon the soft tissues required to form papillae on each side of the implant-supported restoration (Figs 14 – 15).

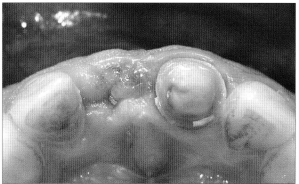

Fig 11   Soft-tissue condition 6 weeks after implant placement.

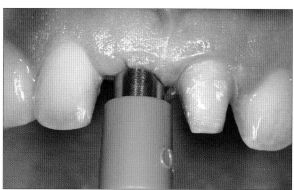

Fig 14   Access surgery to the implant using a 5-mm tissue punch.

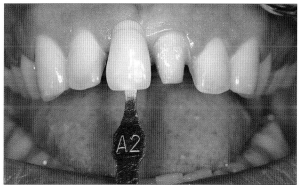

Fig 12   Recording of the appropriate shade for the fabrication of the implant-supported provisional and definitive restorations.

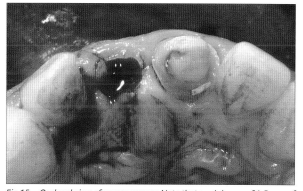

Fig 15   Occlusal view of access surgery. Note that a minimum of 1.5 mm of soft tissue was preserved adjacent to the neighboring teeth and the palatal positioning of the incision.

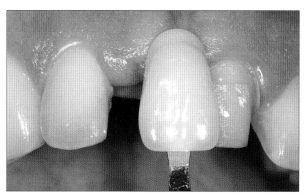

Fig 13   Close-up of the shade tab to record the surface texture and form of adjacent teeth.

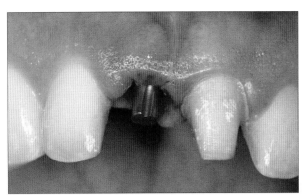

Fig 16   The placement of the temporary 4-mm solid abutment.

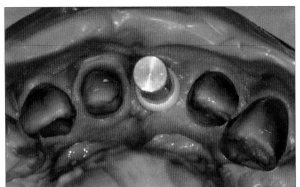

Fig 17   Polyvinyl siloxane impression of the implant shoulder, temporary solid abutment, and adjacent tooth preparation.

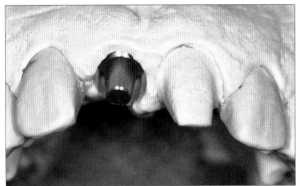

Fig 18   The dental cast to be used for the fabrication of the provisional restoration.

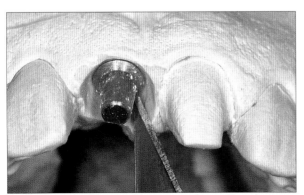

Fig 19   Developing the appropriate emergence form on the cast.

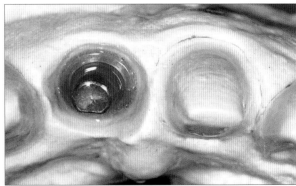

Fig 20   Final outline of the emergence profile for the provisional restoration and the application of the separating medium.

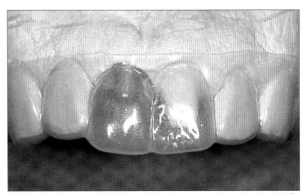

Fig 21   Vacuform matrix fabricated from the diagnostic waxing checked for adaptation.

A 4-mm solid abutment was then positioned and torqued to 15 Ncm. The solid abutment was planned to support the provisional restoration on the implant, and would be removed to allow the placement of the definitive restoration (Fig 16).

An impression cap and positioning cylinder were placed, and a polyvinyl siloxane impression of the implant shoulder, abutment, and adjacent tooth preparation was made (Fig 17). A cast was then poured in rapid-set type 4 dental stone (Fig 18). The cast was modified to provide an estimation of the appropriate emergence form for the provisional restoration, and a separating medium applied. A vacuform matrix of the diagnostic waxing was used to facilitate the fabrication of the implant-supported acrylic-resin provisional prosthesis (Figs 19–22). The finished provisional restoration was then positioned and luted with temporary dental cement (Fig 23).

The patient was re-evaluated after four weeks of healing. The soft tissues were considered healthy. The form and condition of the interproximal tissues were also considered satisfactory (Figs 24–25). The temporary solid abutment was then removed (Fig 26), and a customized syn-Octa impression made of the implant and the sulcus adjacent to it.

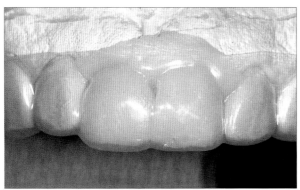

Fig 22   Indirect fabrication of the implant-supported provisional restoration.

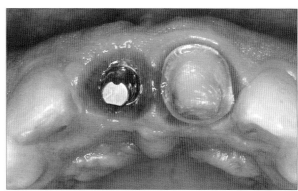

Fig 25   Occlusal view of the sulcus adjacent to the implant after 4 weeks of healing.

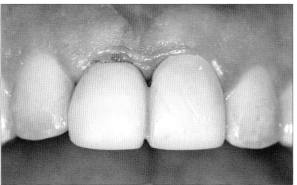

Fig 23   Positioning of the implant-supported and retained provisional fixed dental prosthesis.

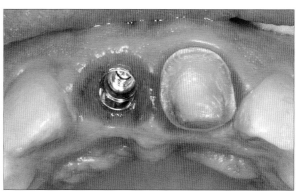

Fig 26   Anterior view of the implant and adjacent teeth after 4 weeks of healing.

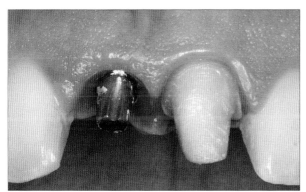

Fig 24   Anterior view of the implant, the temporary abutment and the adjacent teeth after 4 weeks of healing.

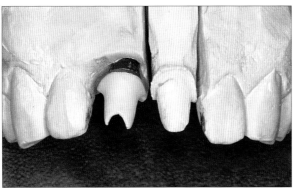

Fig 27   Anterior cast view of the customized metal-ceramic abutment.

The impression was poured in low-expansion type IV dental stone and articulated using appropriate records. A customized metal ceramic abutment was then fabricated using a modified synOcta gold abutment (Figs 27 – 28). This abutment provided a cement line approximately 1 mm apical to the recorded gingival margin, and an increased depth of ceramic in the subgingival region. This would decrease the likelihood of metal reflection through the facial soft tissues subsequent to the placement of the final restoration. The definitive all-ceramic (InCeram) crowns for the central incisors were then fabricated (Fig 29).

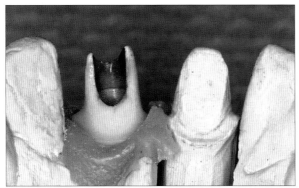

Fig 28   Palatal cast view of the customized metal-ceramic abutment.

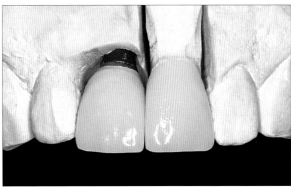

Fig 29   Definitive all-ceramic (InCeram) crowns on the cast.

The customized synOcta gold abutment was tried in intra-orally to confirm the submucosal location of the cement margin and the appropriate support for the interproximal tissues (Fig 30). The definitive crowns were positioned and the proximal contacts and occlusion adjusted as necessary. The adjusted surfaces of the crowns were finished to a glaze-like surface using impregnated disks. The crowns were luted to place with permanent cement, and contacts and occlusion were verified (Figs 31 – 32). At the 3-year follow-up, the patient reported complete satisfaction with the treatment. All tissues appeared to be healthy, and no radiographic abnormality was detected (Fig 33).

Acknowledgments

Laboratory Procedures
Jim Mitchell – M & M Dental Laboratory, Gainesville, Florida, USA.

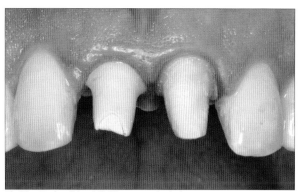

Fig 30   Try-in of the definitive customized abutment.

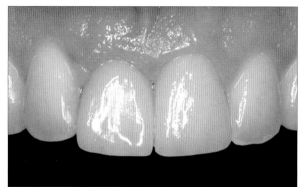

Fig 31   Anterior view. The final all-ceramic restorations in position.

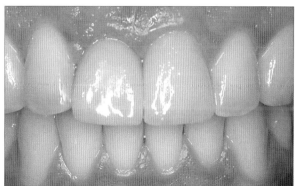

Fig 32   Anterior view. Maximum intercuspation of definitive all-ceramic restorations.

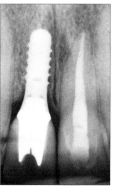

Fig 33   Radiograph taken at the 3-year follow-up.

4.13 Replacement of a Maxillary Right Central Incisor Using an Early Loading Protocol

J. Ganeles

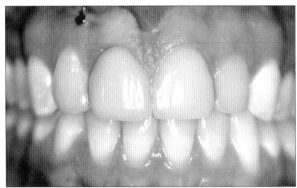

Fig 1   Initial presentation.

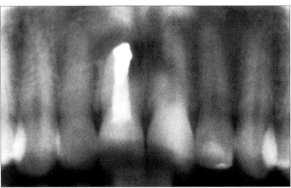

Fig 2   Pre-treatment radiograph.

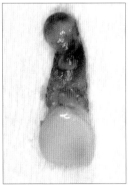

Fig 3   Extracted tooth with periapical granuloma.

A healthy 26-year-old woman was referred for evaluation and treatment of her failing maxillary right central incisor (tooth 11). She reportedly traumatized the tooth at about age 9 and subsequently had repeated conventional and surgical endodontic procedures and fixed restorations. Despite these procedures, she had recurrent fistulas in the apical mucosa and a mid-facial pocket of 7 mm with suppuration (Fig 1). All other sites on the tooth probed 3 mm without inflammation.

She presented with a medium biotype with triangularly-shaped teeth and a moderately high smile line, showing all of her papillas and a few millimeters of marginal gingiva in a full smile. Ceramic veneers were present on teeth 12, 21, and 22, and they were known to be somewhat bulky, eventually requiring replacement. She had a strong desire to avoid additional tooth preparation and would not consider a fixed dental prosthesis to replace tooth 11.

The rest of her dentition was intact restoratively, occlusally, and periodontally. Periapical and orthopantomographic radiographs indicated a large periapical radiolucency on tooth 11, without other pathology (Fig 2). An endodontist evaluated the tooth and suspected an apical root fracture or other untreatable periapical pathology, giving tooth 11 a hopeless prognosis. Bone levels on the adjacent teeth appeared normal, without crestal resorption.

After the relevant conversations and obtaining informed consent, tooth 11 was extracted without raising a flap (Fig 3). The socket was thoroughly curetted to ensure the complete removal of the apical granuloma and other soft tissue. A collagen sponge was placed into the socket to aid in hemostasis. At the same appointment, a temporary removable partial denture was inserted and adjusted to provide cosmetic replacement for the tooth, without placing significant pressure on the marginal tissues.

After 5 weeks of uneventful healing, the patient returned for implant surgery. Upon reexamination, significant collapse of the buccal contour was evident (Figs 4a – d).

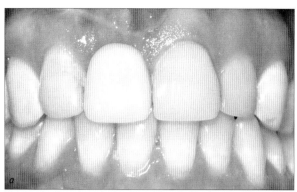

Figs 4a – d   5 weeks post-extraction with and without removable provisional appliance showing collapse of tissue.

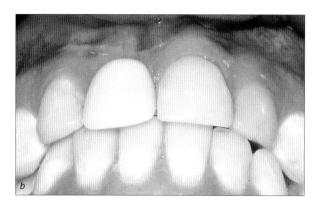

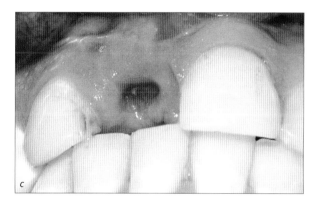

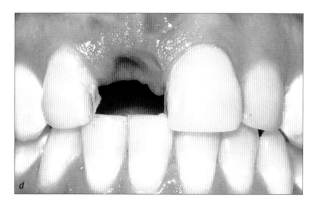

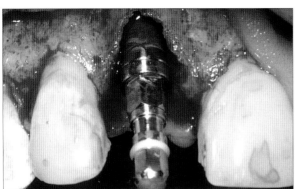

Fig 5a   Regular Neck implant with carrier attached after seating to proper three-dimensional position, anterior view.

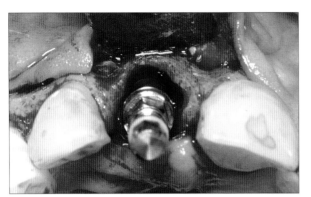

Fig 5b   Regular Neck implant with carrier attached after seating to proper three-dimensional position, occlusal view.

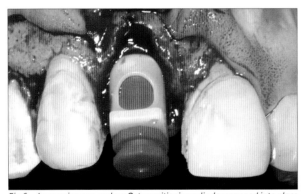

Fig 6   Impression cap and synOcta positioning cylinder snapped into place prior to suturing.

Implant surgery was performed with simultaneous bone augmentation after the reflection of full thickness flaps. The socket was again thoroughly curetted and implant osteotomy performed, anticipating the ideal three-dimensional position of the implant. A Straumann Standard Plus implant (endosteal diameter, 4.1 mm, length, 12 mm, Regular Neck prosthetic platform, 4.8 mm) with SLA surface was seated to a position centered between the adjacent teeth, approximately 2 mm apical to the cemento-enamel junction of tooth 21 with the central axis tilted just palatal to the anticipated incisal edge of the final restoration (Figs 5a – b).

As the implant was seated at approximately 25 Ncm of insertion torque, a transfer impression was taken to facilitate the future provisional preparation. To accomplish this, a synOcta impression cap and positioning cylinder were attached to the implant. Subsequently, a full-arch polyvinylsiloxane (PVS) impression was made after protecting the implant surface from the impression material (Fig 6).

Following the transfer, a large healing cap was placed on the implant. Autogenous bone and connective tissue were harvested from the right tuberosity area. Bone chips were condensed over the facially dehisced areas of the implant with an attempt to completely correct the defect area, overcompensating in height and width at the buccoocclusal line angle area. This graft was covered with a resorbable collagen membrane (Fig 7). De-epithelialized gingival connective tissue, harvested as a distal wedge, was positioned over the bone graft and secured with resorbable sutures. The overlying flaps were advanced using periosteal releasing incisions and sutured over the grafted site, obtaining primary closure and providing an optimal submerged healing environment for the hard and soft tissue grafts (Fig 8). The patient's temporary removable denture was relieved gingivally to avoid pressure on the surgical site.

During the healing period, the surgical impression, records, opposing-cast, and shade information were sent to the dental technician for the fabrication of a screw-retained provisional restoration (Fig 9). A synOcta titanium provisional cylinder served as the core of the restoration, with composite as the esthetic material. Crown contours were created to harmonize with the adjacent teeth, while root contours were developed to harmonize the subgingival transition from the implant to the coronal form.

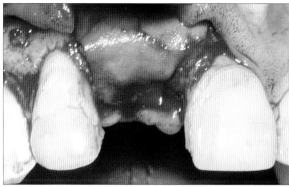

Fig 7   Implant submerged under resorbable collagen membrane after bone grafting.

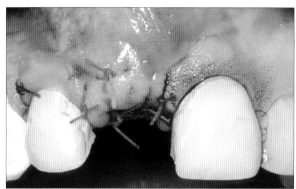

Fig 8   Flaps advanced and sutured after addition of gingival connective tissue graft.

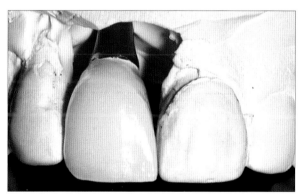

Figs 9   Screw-retained composite provisional restoration fabricated on analog model.

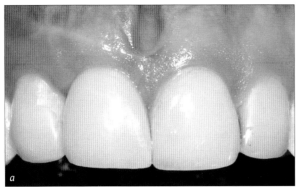

Figs 10a – b   Provisional restoration seated after implant exposure.

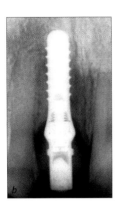

Ten weeks following implant surgery, the implant was un-covered to attach the provisional restoration and begin tissue contouring. The implant was exposed and facial tis-sue additionally augmented using a "roll technique" in which gingiva coronal to the closure screw was incised proximally and palatally, de-epithelialized, then purse-string sutured apically under the facial gingiva. The pur-pose of this technique was to additionally augment the fa-cial gingiva, recreating a root eminence. The prefabricat-ed provisional restoration was seated with screw retention (Figs 10a – b). Blanching of the surrounding gingiva was observed, but soon diminished.

Two months following the provisional placement, after gingival healing and minor contour modification, final im-pressions were taken. A soft-tissue transfer technique was used to communicate gingival contours to the dental technician (Figs 11a – b).

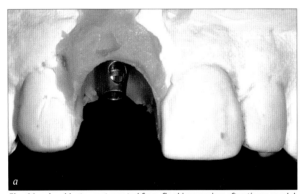

Figs 11a – b   Master cast created from final impression after tissue model-ing and transfer of gingival contours.

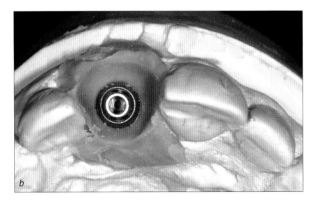

It was decided that a metal-ceramic restoration with transversal screw retention would be the most appropriate restorative design for this situation for several reasons. First, the subgingival depth of the margins palatally and interproximally dictated that screw retention was indicated. Second, the observation that the axis channel (screw emergence) was near the incisal edge made it difficult to control esthetic materials using a standard screw-retained restoration. Finally, the patient's high smile line and esthetic demands created the desire to apply ceramic material to the implant margin to optimize optical properties of the site and provide light reflection and gingival illumination subgingivally. Given these desires and constraints, the dental technician created a metal ceramic restoration using synOcta transversal (TS) components (Figs 12a – c).

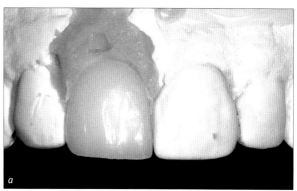

Figs 12a – c   Metal-ceramic restoration with transversal screw (TS) retention on master cast.

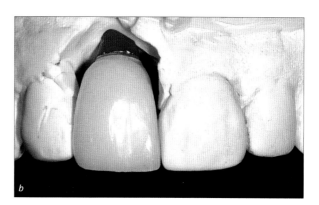

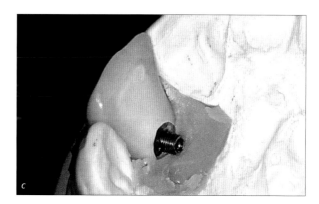

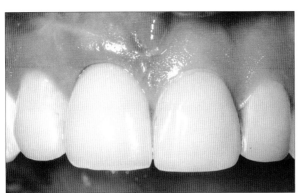

Fig 13   Appearance four weeks following the insertion of the final restoration.

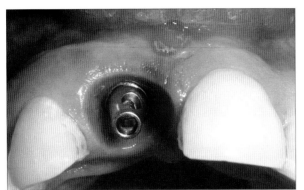

Fig 14   Healthy subgingival contours four weeks following the insertion of the final restoration.

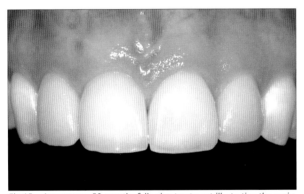

Fig 15   Appearance 50 months following treatment illustrating the maintenance of gingival stability.

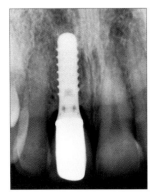

Figs 16   Radiograph 50 months following treatment illustrating maintenance of crestal stability.

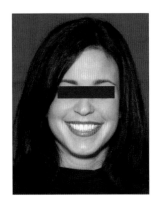

Figs 17   Excellent esthetics at 50-month evaluation.

The final restoration was delivered approximately 8 weeks after final impressions. About 4 weeks following insertion, the patient returned for evaluation and to check gingival response (Fig 13). For photographic purposes, the restoration was removed (Fig 14). Excellent esthetics and gingival symmetry tissue responses were observed. Of particular interest was the maintenance of the healthy subgingival transition area, which appeared completely epithelialized without inflammation. Also noteworthy was the maintenance of the buccal/gingival volume and form, and the appearance of a "root eminence" for tooth 11.

Two years later, the patient had the ceramic veneers on the other maxillary incisors replaced. She was followed up for approximately two more years and returned for periodic evaluation at 50 months. At that visit, clinical, photographic, and radiographic evaluations were performed (Figs 15 – 17). Gingival health, dimensional stability, and superb esthetics were maintained. Excellent symmetry of the marginal gingiva of tooth 11 was seen when compared to tooth 21. Nearly identical papilla heights were observed when comparing sites 11 – 12 with sites 21 – 22. This represented an improvement in papilla height between teeth 12 and 11 as compared to the early post-insertion photographs. The radiograph showed the normal crestal-bone remodeling around the implant that is expected with Straumann implants. Normal bone-implant radiographic appearance can be observed around the rest of the implant. Interproximal bone heights were maintained on the adjacent teeth.

For photographic purposes, the implant crown was removed to evaluate the peri-implant gingival interface (Figs 18a – b). The tissue appearance was very similar to the early post-insertion photos with the maintenance of an epithelialized sulcus, excellent tissue health, and dimensional stability. The papillae at the adjacent teeth were formed normally. Close inspection of the sulcus suggests the formation of vascular loops in the subgingival tissue, confirming the lack of visible inflammation.

In conclusion, this case demonstrates the replacement of a chronically infected central incisor in a moderately damaged alveolar ridge in a patient with high esthetic demands. The procedures used were selected for maximum efficacy and predictability to rebuild and regenerate lost alveolar tissues in conjunction with implant placement. Additionally, by anticipating and planning restorative procedures with a surgical implant impression, treatment time was greatly reduced and gingival contouring was significantly accelerated. This allowed the dental laboratory to create a provisional restoration for placement at the implant uncovering appointment, dramatically reducing the need for tissue-conditioning adjustments and appointments. The excellent esthetics at the long-term follow-up clearly demonstrate the stability of the implant, the restoration, and the surrounding tissue.

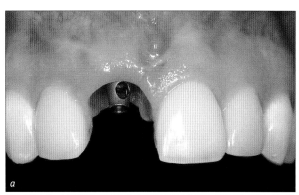

Figs 18a – b   Healthy subgingival contours without inflammation at 50-month evaluation.

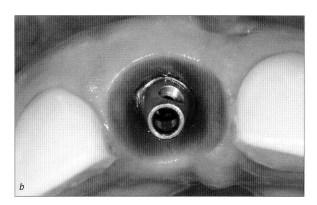

Acknowledgments
Dr. Joel Gale – Aventura, Florida, USA, for ceramic veneer restorations.

Laboratory Procedures
Michael Hahn – DAS Dentallabor, Boca Raton, Florida, USA, for all restorations shown.

Multi-Tooth Gaps in the Anterior Maxilla

4.14 Replacement of the Four Maxillary Incisors with a Fixed Dental Prosthesis Using an Immediate Loading Protocol

D. Morton, J. Ruskin

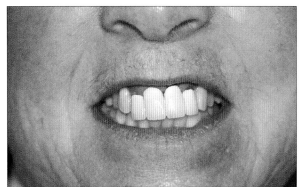

Fig 1   Pre-treatment anterior profile.

In November 2001, a 53-year-old female presented seeking advice and options for treatment of her maxillary incisor teeth. She was dissatisfied with both the functional and esthetic qualities of her existing restorations (Figs 1 – 3). Her medical health was excellent, and she reported no contraindications to dental care.

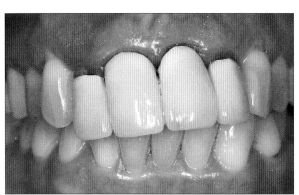

Fig 2   Pre-treatment retracted anterior view. Maximum intercuspation.

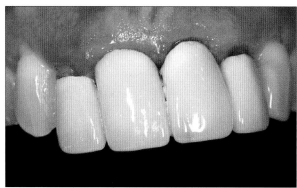

Fig 3   Pre-treatment retracted anterior view. Maxillary restorations.

On presentation, the patient's dental health was less than ideal. Although she had no probing depths greater than 3 mm, she suffered from generalized chronic adult periodontitis and displayed multiple sites of bleeding on probing. Her remaining dentition was heavily restored, and many teeth had been endodontically treated. Areas of recurrent dental caries were noted on many teeth. Radiographically and clinically, the maxillary incisor teeth exhibited large areas of active caries (Figs 4 – 7), and after the splinted crowns had been removed, the teeth were determined to be non-restorable. Subsequent to caries removal, a provisional restoration was placed and the patient was referred to the Departments of Periodontology and Operative Dentistry for disease-control procedures.

Adequate space must be maintained between implants and teeth and between adjacent implants. A detailed evaluation of the patient's anterior maxilla indicated insufficient room for four implants (1.5 mm between implants and teeth and 3 mm between implants). The decision, therefore, was to plan for two dental implants and a four-unit fixed dental prosthesis. Several options were considered with regard to implant position. These included:

- Option 1: Placement of two implants in the central incisor sites.
- Option 2: Placement of two implants in the lateral incisor sites.
- Option 3: Placement of two staggered implants, one in a central incisor site, and the other in the contralateral lateral incisor site.

The placement of two implants in the central incisor regions had advantages. This placement option was thought to maximize the bone-implant contact using standard diameter implants (4.1 mm) that could be ideally positioned with regard to planned restorations. In addition, options were available for both the provisional and the definitive restorative phases of treatment (cement and screw retention). Disadvantages included the need for adjacent implants, although the realistic esthetic demands of the patient and the moderate to thick tissue biotype minimized this concern.

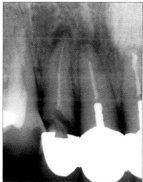 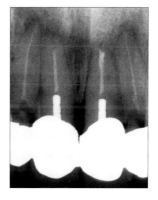 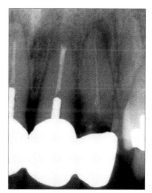

Figs 4 – 6   Pre-treatment periapical radiographs, maxillary incisors.

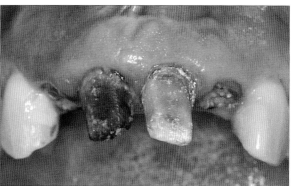

Fig 7   Pre-treatment retracted anterior view. Maxillary incisor teeth.

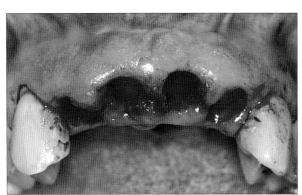

Fig 8   Anterior maxilla subsequent to tooth extraction.

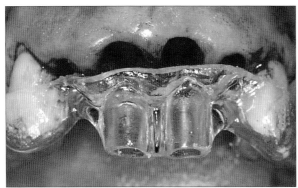

Fig 9   Surgical template in place. This template was designed to guide the mesiodistal and orofacial positioning of the implants.

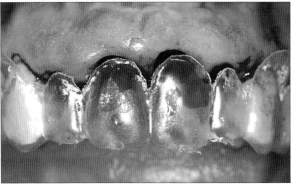

Fig 10   Depth template in place. This template was designed to communicate the desired implant shoulder (restorative margin) depth.

The placement of two implants in the lateral incisor sites was not considered appropriate, as restoration-driven implant placement encroached upon the neighboring teeth.

Although her esthetic expectations were realistic, the patient was concerned about her appearance throughout the healing phase. With this in mind, she was given treatment alternatives. These included:

- Extraction of the teeth, followed by a period of healing prior to the placement of the implants. During this period, an interim removable partial prosthesis would be worn. Implants would be positioned subsequent to ridge healing.
- Extraction of the teeth, followed by immediate (type 1) placement of two implants in the central incisor sites, should conditions be favorable.

The patient was also given options with regard to the interim restoration of the missing incisors subsequent to implant placement. These included:

- Use of an interim removable partial prosthesis until the loading of the implants (6 – 8 weeks) with a provisional restoration.
- Immediate loading of the implants with an acrylic-resin provisional fixed prosthesis.

After considering her options, the patient consented to treatment and elected to proceed with the following plan:

- Extraction of the teeth.
- If the conditions were favorable (maintenance of facial bone and minimum trauma to the soft tissues), immediate placement of the dental implants in the central incisor sites would be undertaken.
- Should the implants exhibit adequate stability, then the immediate loading (provisional restoration in contact with opposing dentition) of the implants with a four-unit provisional fixed dental prosthesis would be undertaken.

The patient was advised of the risk of complication associated with the proposed plans. Risks included early implant loss with possible destruction of the implant sites and the consequent need for grafting and longer treatment times. She was also advised of the necessity to minimize any functional contact on the immediate provisional restoration.

The maxillary incisor teeth (12 – 22) were removed with a minimum of trauma to hard and soft tissues (Fig 8), and the central incisor sites were considered adequate for the immediate (Type 1) placement of implants. Surgical templates (Figs 9 – 11) were used to prepare the sites according to the planned restorations, and two Straumann Tapered Effect (TE) implants (endosteal diameter, 4.1 mm; length, 10 mm; Regular Neck prosthetic platform, 4.8 mm) were positioned and considered stable (Fig 12). Two 4-mm solid abutments were chosen to support the provisional restorations and positioned with 15 Ncm of torque (Fig 13).

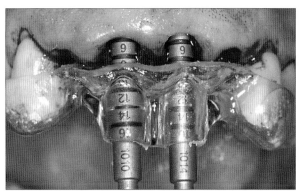

Fig 11 Confirmation of osteotomy inclination in the mesiodistal and orofacial directions.

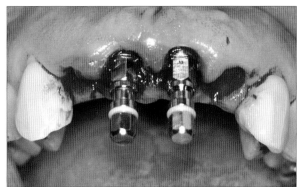

Fig 12 Positioning of the two Straumann Tapered Effect implants.

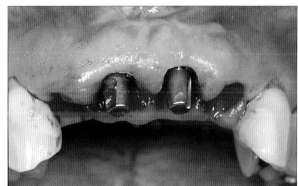

Fig 13 Positioning of the temporary (4 mm) abutments, anterior view.

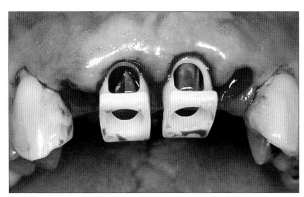

Fig 14   Placement of the impression caps.

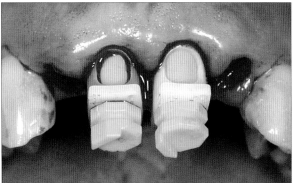

Fig 15   Placement of the positioning cylinders.

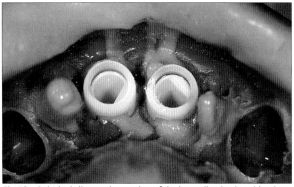

Fig 16   Polyvinyl siloxane impression of the immediately placed implants and abutments.

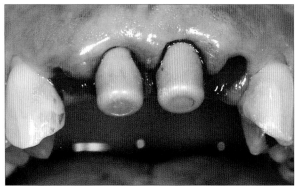

Fig 17   Protective caps in position to prevent tissue collapse.

Impression caps and positioning cylinders (for 4-mm solid abutments) were carefully placed (Figs 14–15), and a polyvinyl siloxane impression was made to record the position of the implants and remaining teeth (Fig 16). Protective caps were positioned onto the abutments to prevent tissue collapse during the fabrication of the provisional restorations in the laboratory (Fig 17).

Indirect fabrication of the provisional fixed prosthesis was considered to be less traumatic to the implant sites compared to the direct alternatives. Impression-making was considered a safe treatment procedure due to the implant's stability. An inability on the part of the implants to tolerate impression procedures would have been considered a contraindication to immediate loading.

Implant analogs were then positioned into the impression, which was poured in low-expansion type IV dental stone (Figs 18 – 19). The stone cast was modified to provide ovate pontic form in the regions of the lateral incisors, and appropriate emergence around the implants. A separating medium was applied to the cast (Fig 20). The provisional restorations were then fabricated on the cast and finished.

The provisional restoration was adjusted intraorally to provide stable occlusal contacts in maximum intercuspation and minimize contacts in excursive movements, particularly protrusion. It was then polished and luted with polycarboxylate cement (Figs 21 – 22). A radiograph was obtained as the post-surgical baseline and to confirm the appropriate position of the implants. The occlusal conditions were verified, and the careful control of load was reiterated to the patient.

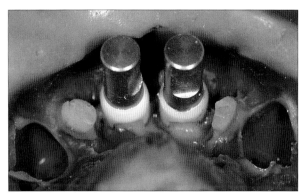

Fig 18   Positioning of the implant analogs in the impression.

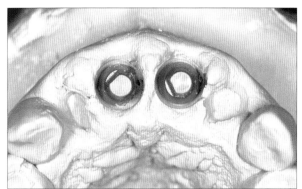

Fig 19   Low expansion type IV dental stone cast for the indirect fabrication of the provisional restorations.

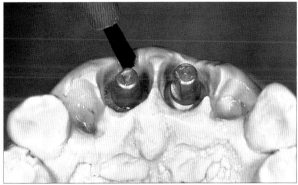

Fig 20   Application of separating medium to the modified cast. The cast was altered to provide ovate pontic form for the lateral incisors.

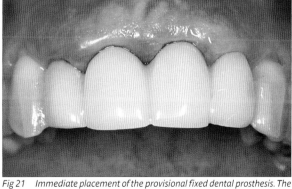

Fig 21   Immediate placement of the provisional fixed dental prosthesis. The prosthesis was characterized by central incisor retainers and cantilevered ovate pontics in the lateral incisor regions.

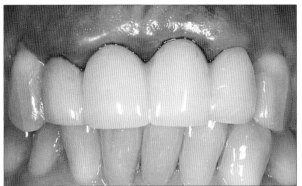

Fig 22   The immediately positioned provisional fixed dental prosthesis.

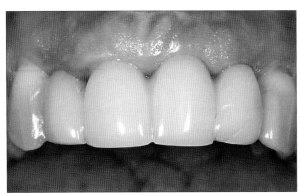

Fig 23 Provisional fixed dental prosthesis 12 weeks after implant placement, anterior view.

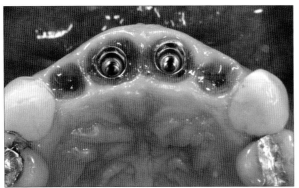

Fig 24 Occlusal view of soft tissues 12 weeks after implant placement.

The patient was seen for follow-up at intervals of 1, 4, and 8 weeks. She described only minimal postoperative discomfort, and at no time did the provisional restoration appear or feel loose. The provisional restoration and tissue response were evaluated 12 weeks subsequent to the implant placement (Fig 23). The conditions were considered favorable for the making of the final impressions. The provisional restoration and temporary abutments were removed and the implant shoulders cleaned of cement residue (Fig 24).

The provisional restoration was then cleaned of residual cement and implant and abutment duplicates were positioned. The provisional restoration and duplicates were then embedded into firm-set polyvinyl siloxane registration material to a depth of the proximal contacts (Figs 25 – 26). After the setting of the registration material, the provisional restoration was removed to reveal a duplication of the transition zone (or submucosal profile) from the restorative margin of the implant to the free gingival margin (Fig 27).

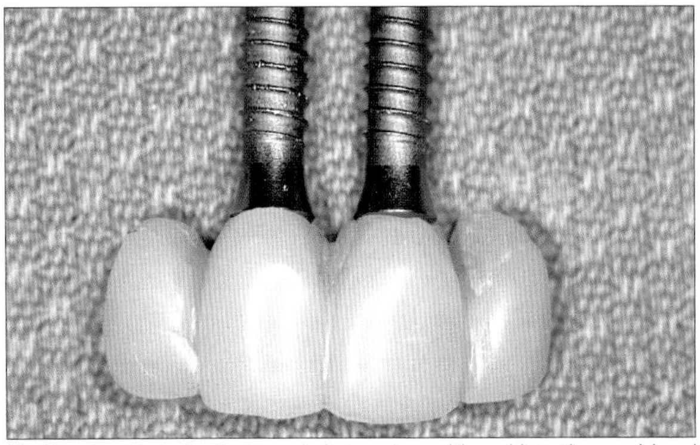

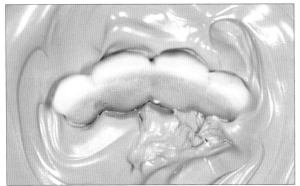

Fig 25 Duplicate implants and abutments positioned into the provisional prosthesis.

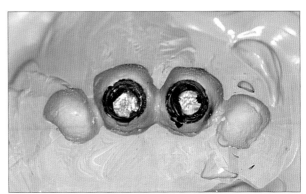

Fig 26 Duplicates and provisional restoration embedded in registration material to the depth of the proximal contacts.

Fig 27 Duplication of the submucosal emergence profile established intraorally by the provisional restoration.

Impression caps and positioning cylinders were then carefully placed onto the embedded implant and abutment duplicates (Figs 28 – 29). Autopolymerizing acrylic resin was then introduced into the space around the impression caps and into the ovate pontic regions to duplicate the form of the provisional restoration (Fig 30).

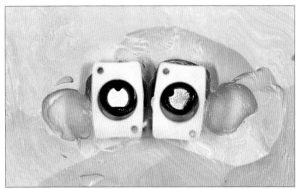
Fig 28   Impression caps positioned onto the implant duplicates.

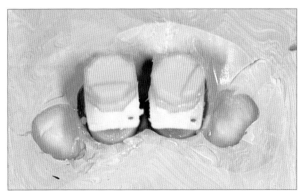
Fig 29   Positioning cylinders placed into the impression caps.

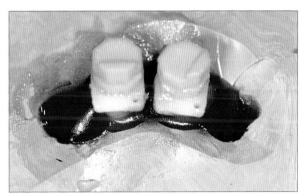
Fig 30   Autopolymerizing acrylic resin placed into the space surrounding the implants and the ovate pontic sites.

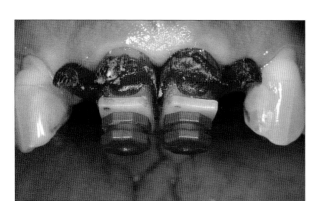

Fig 31   Customized impression caps and synOcta positioning cylinders in place.

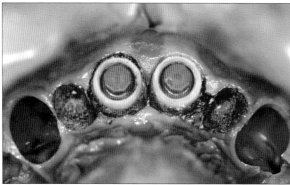

Fig 32   Final polyvinyl siloxane impression incorporating the customized impression copings. The acrylic resin duplicated the emergence profile developed by the provisional restoration.

The customized impression caps were positioned onto the implants and synOcta positioning cylinders were placed to record the implant timing (Fig 31). An impression of the maxillary arch was then obtained using polyvinyl siloxane impression material (Fig 32). The master cast was then poured in low-expansion dental stone and synOcta Transversal (TS) abutments positioned to support the planned restoration. The master cast duplicated the emergence profile of the provisional retainers in the central incisor sites and the ovate pontic form planned for the lateral incisors.

A screw-retained fixed dental prosthesis was planned to eliminate the possibility of residual cement entrapment at the time of the definitive prosthesis delivery. A framework was waxed, cast, and verified for occlusal clearance and passivity (Figs 33 – 35). Dental ceramic was then fused to the framework in sequential layers to provide for the planned shade and tooth contour (Figs 36 – 37). The passivity of the final prosthesis was verified on the cast prior to its return from the laboratory.

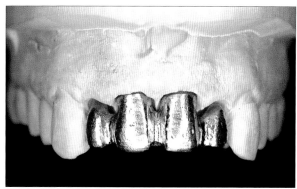

Fig 33   Anterior view of the definitive framework.

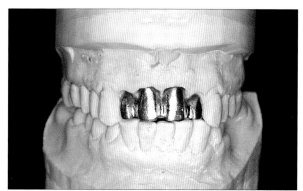

Fig 34   Framework in position on articulated casts to verify adequate room for the addition of dental ceramic.

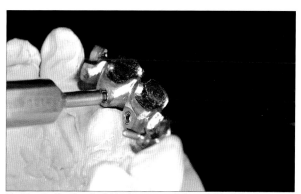

Fig 35   Verification (individual screw passivity and fit) of the framework passivity.

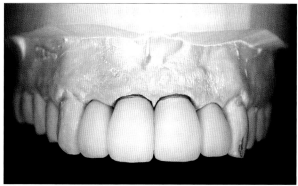

Fig 36   Anterior view of the completed fixed dental prosthesis.

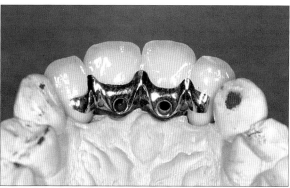

Fig 37   Palatal view of the completed fixed dental prosthesis.

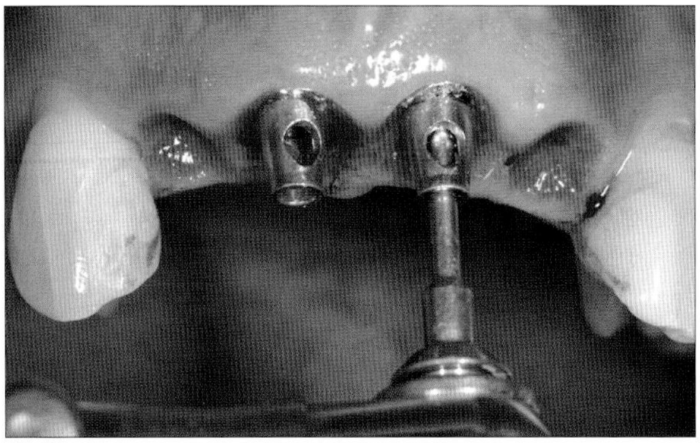

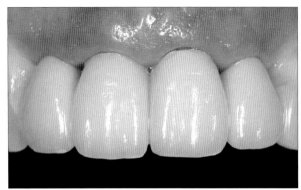

Fig 38   Torquing of the definitive synOcta TS abutments.

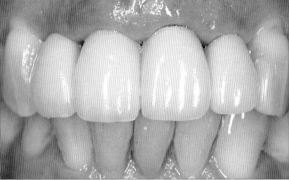

Fig 39   The positioning of the final prosthesis. Note the exposed metal margin on the facial aspect of the left central incisor. The soft tissues adjacent to the right central incisor and the ovate pontic sites were considered excellent.

At the delivery appointment, the provisional restoration and abutments were removed and the implants cleaned and dried. The health and form of the surrounding soft tissues was confirmed. The synOcta TS abutments were positioned and torqued to 35 Ncm without incident and the definitive restoration positioned and lightly screwed to place to confirm seating (Figs 38 – 39). Occlusal and proximal contacts were verified and adjusted, and the restoration polished as required prior to the finger-pressure tightening of the transversal screws.

Although the patient was completely satisfied with the esthetic outcome, it can be noted that the metal margin of the restoration was visible on the implant in the position of tooth 21 (Figs 39 – 40). Probing revealed a sulcus depth of approximately 1 mm on the facial aspect, and the decision was made to evaluate the tissue response after 6 weeks of service.

Fig 40   Anterior view of the final prosthesis in maximum intercuspation.

D. Morton, J. Ruskin

At the 6-week review appointment, the exposed metal margin had been submerged by the repositioning or coronal migration of the surrounding soft tissues (Fig 41). A radiograph confirmed satisfactory maintenance of bone in the regions of the ovate pontics and between the implants (Fig 42). After three years of service, the prosthesis and all tissues remained healthy (Fig 43), and the patient was completely satisfied with all aspects of the treatment.

Acknowledgments

Laboratory Procedures

Todd A. Fridrich – Definitive Dental Arts, Coralville, Iowa, USA.

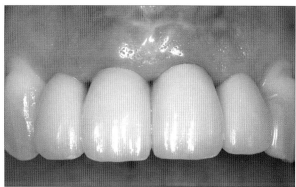

Fig 41   Anterior view of the prosthesis after six weeks of service. Note the coronal rebound of the facial soft tissues surrounding the left central retainer.

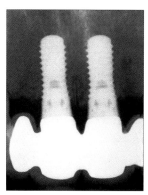

Fig 42   Radiograph made at the 6-week post-delivery follow-up.

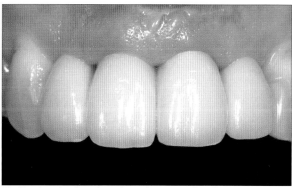

Fig 43   Anterior view of prostheses three years after placement.

4.15 Replacement of the Four Maxillary Incisors with a Fixed Dental Prosthesis Using an Early Loading Protocol

S. Chen, A. Dickinson

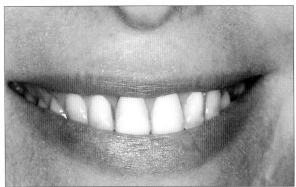

Fig 1   Extraoral frontal view, showing the patient's smile.

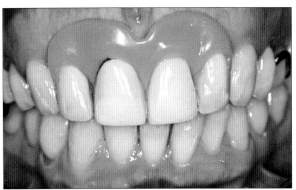

Fig 2   Intraoral frontal view, showing an acrylic upper partial denture with a large flange replacing the four missing upper incisors (teeth 12, 11, 21, and 22).

In March 2004, a 46-year-old female patient presented, seeking options to replace her existing acrylic maxillary removable partial denture, which replaced the four maxillary incisor teeth. She had been wearing this partial denture for approximately 15 years, the teeth having been extracted when the patient was in her early twenties. She did not want a further removable prosthesis as she was unhappy with the appearance of the flange on the denture. She was interested in exploring options for a fixed solution as long as the esthetic outcomes were not adverse.

The patient was in good health, with no systemic contraindications to implant therapy. She had good oral hygiene and was a well-motivated individual with sound natural teeth and healthy periodontal support.

An extraoral examination revealed a normal physiognomy and normal facial and lip support. On full smiling, the gingival margins of the upper teeth were just visible (Fig 1). At the intraoral examination, a removable partial denture was noted, replacing teeth 12, 11, 21, and 22 (Fig 2). The denture carried a large and thick acrylic labial flange.

An assessment of the edentulous region revealed a well-formed ridge with good buccal contour and ridge height (Figs 3 – 4). The mucosa was thick with a wide zone of keratinized mucosa. The tissue biotype was thick. In addition to the four maxillary incisors, tooth 28 was missing (Fig 5).

Plain film tomography showed the presence of a relatively thin ridge in the horizontal plane, with sufficient vertical height (Fig 6). The apparently thick contour of the ridge was due to the presence of a thick mucosa orally and facially. A slight concavity on the buccal aspect of the bony ridge was noted. The orofacial bone width was estimated to be approximately 4 – 5 mm.

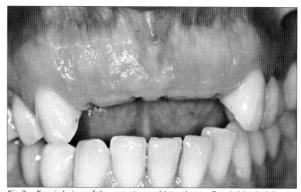

Fig 3   Frontal view of the anterior multi-tooth gap. Good ridge height was noted.

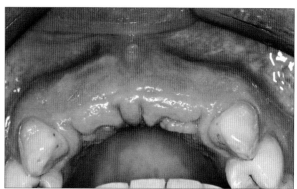

Fig 4   Occlusal view, showing the ridge with what appeared to be adequate horizontal ridge width.

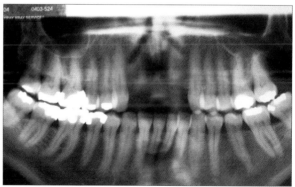

Fig 5   Orthopantomogram of the patient's dentition at the time of presentation.

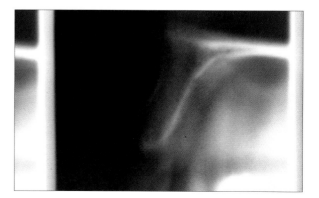

Fig 6   Plain film tomogram of the maxillary anterior ridge, showing a relatively thin ridge in the horizontal plane. The apparent ridge thickness was due to thick mucosa at the crestal and oral surfaces.

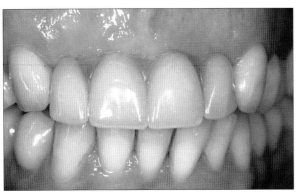

Fig 7   Frontal view of the try-in of a diagnostic denture. The denture was fabricated without a flange. The image shows that the existing ridge volume appeared to be adequate to achieve a good esthetic result without a denture flange. In order to achieve a good soft-tissue esthetic result, implant placement congruent with the cervical margins of the planned prosthetic lateral incisor teeth is required. The lateral incisors are relatively small (mesiodistally) which will demand implant placement in close proximity to each adjacent canine.

Following discussions with the patient on her esthetic demands, the relative lack of horizontal bone width, and the presence of a thick acrylic flange on the denture that was providing lip support, she agreed to undertake a diagnostic phase. Impressions were obtained, and a diagnostic removable acrylic denture without a flange was constructed. This was delivered to the patient to evaluate lip support, gingival esthetics, and phonetics (Figs 7 – 8). The patient took the denture away with her, and returned a week later expressing satisfaction with the appearance of the prosthesis.

A CT scan was then obtained with the patient wearing a custom radiographic stent for computer-assisted navigational surgery (Image Guided Implants IGI, DenX, Melbourne, Australia) (Fig 9). The number, location, and axial orientation of implants were determined on reformatted cross-sectional images using the IGI planning software program (Figs 10 – 16). The treatment plan was to place two Straumann Standard Plus Narrow Neck (NN) implants at sites 12 and 22 for the construction of a four-unit fixed dental prosthesis.

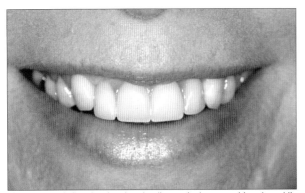

Fig 8   Frontal view showing that the diagnostic denture achieved good lip support, and acceptable facial and dental esthetics.

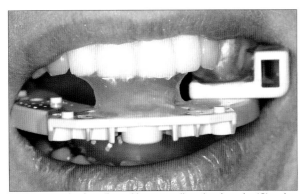

Fig 9   The try-in of a radiographic stent to allow planning using IGI navigational software (DenX, Melbourne, Australia).

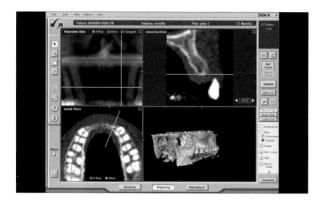
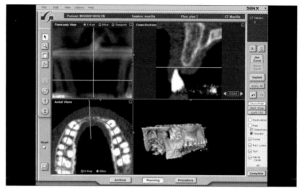
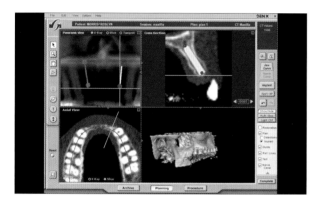
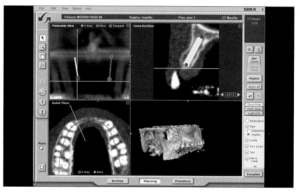
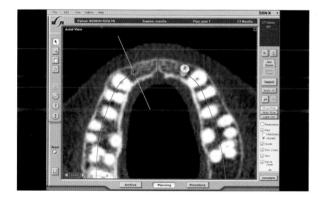
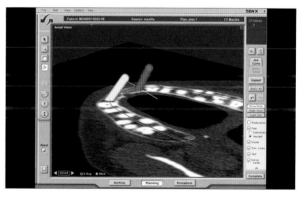

Figs 10–16   *Preoperative assessment of the CT scans and planning using the IGI software confirmed that the best sites for implants were the lateral incisor regions. The treatment plan was to precisely position two implants in the position of the planned prosthetic lateral incisor teeth using IGI software. The implants would be used to support a four-unit fixed dental prosthesis. Due to the relatively narrow dimensions of the lateral incisors, and narrow orofacial dimensions of the ridge, the implants chosen were Narrow Neck implants. The images show the plan to place two Straumann Standard Plus implants with Narrow Neck prosthetic platform (endosteal diameter, 3.3 mm, length, 12 mm, Narrow Neck prosthetic platform, 3.5 mm).*

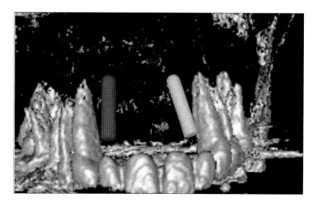

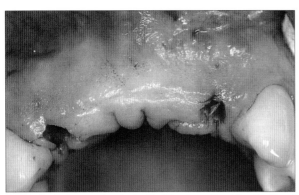

Fig 17   Implants were placed using the IGI system without the elevation of surgical flaps. A small tissue punch was used to remove the mucosa at the implant sites.

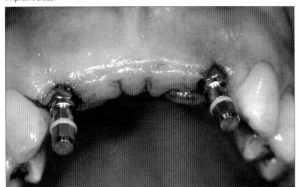

Fig 18   Frontal view of the implants with the transfer parts attached.

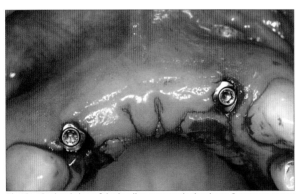

Fig 19   Occlusal view of the healing caps on the implants. Sutures were not required.

In July of 2004, surgery was performed using navigational methods without flap elevation under local anaesthesia (Figs 17 – 19). The correct location of the implants was verified using the diagnostic denture (Figs 20 – 21). The bone was soft in quality. One week later, healing was seen to be progressing well, with no postoperative complications (Fig 22). The integration of the implants was verified at 8 weeks by applying 35 Ncm of torque (Figs 23 – 24). Intraoral periapical radiographs of the implants at this time showed ideal bone conditions (Figs 25 – 26)

Restorative treatment commenced 8 weeks postoperatively. Narrow Neck implant impression copings (directly screw-retained) were placed and an impression was made using a polyvinyl siloxane impression material. A type IV stone master cast was constructed that included removable resilient silicone 'soft tissue' around the necks of the NN laboratory analogs contained within the master cast. A facebow recording, interocclusal record, lower impression, and other esthetic records were obtained.

From a full-contour diagnostic wax-up, individual metal-ceramic mesostructures were fabricated, using standard Straumann framework blanks. These components allow for the direct sintering of ceramic material to their surface following any required structural modification and degassing. The mesostructures were finalized utilizing an opaque ceramic layer fused to the surface of the vertical walls and a ceramic shoulder circumferentially (Figs 27 – 28). The geometry of the shoulder allowed it to follow the natural scalloping of the mucosa around the implant as well as to provide for the placement of a restorative interface for the definitive prosthesis, being approximately 1 – 2 mm submucosal on the labial and proximal aspects.

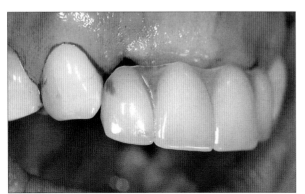
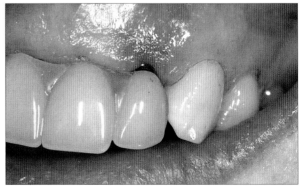

Figs 20 – 21   The verification of the position of the implants in relation to the planned position was confirmed with the diagnostic denture. Note that the healing caps are located immediately subjacent to the lateral incisors in precisely the correct positions.

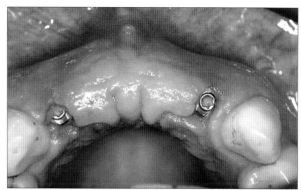

Fig 22 Occlusal view of the surgical sites 1 week postoperatively. The patient was instructed to rinse with a 0.2% solution of chlorhexidine for 1 week. Mechanical plaque removal was instituted 1 week after surgery.

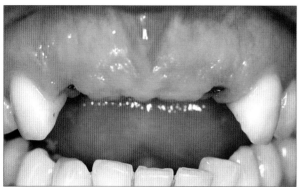

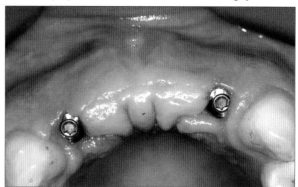

Figs 23 – 24 Frontal and occlusal views of the implant sites after 8 weeks of healing. The implants were successfully integrated.

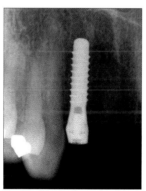

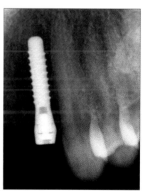

Figs 25 – 26 Radiographs of the implants after 2 months of healing. Note the precise placement adjacent to the upper canines, with sufficient space to avoid trauma to the natural teeth.

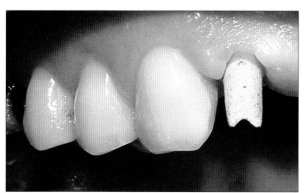

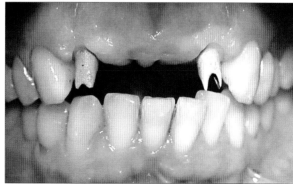

Figs 27 – 28 The try-in of individual metal-ceramic mesostructures that were fabricated using standard components. Ceramic material was directly sintered to the surface and finalized using an opaque ceramic layer fused to the surface of the vertical walls and a ceramic shoulder circumferentially.

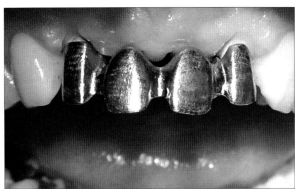

Fig 29   The try-in of the FDP metal framework.

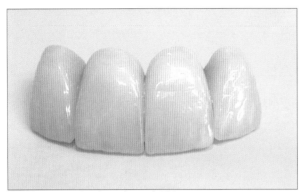

Fig 30   The completed metal-ceramic FDP.

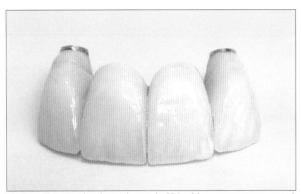

Fig 31   The completed metal-ceramic FDP with mesostructures seated, demonstrating the contour of the transmucosal components.

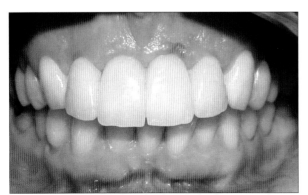

Fig 32   Frontal view of the fixed dental prosthesis after cementation.

The mesostructures were tried in and the fixed dental prosthesis metal framework tested for passive and accurate seating (Fig 29). At that time, the position and circumferential dimensions of the ceramic shoulder were evaluated to ensure that there was desirable displacement of the peri-implant mucosa. The final evaluation of the interarch relationship and framework design was undertaken. The partially fabricated prosthesis was then retrieved, the mesostructures were removed, and the standard beveled healing caps replaced.

The definitive metal-ceramic prosthesis, cemented to the custom-fabricated mesostrucures was placed four weeks following the commencement of the restorative treatment (Figs 30 – 31). The mesostructures were first placed, each with the designated NN auxiliary screw taken to 35 Ncm. The fixed dental prosthesis was cemented to place using a modified glass-ionomer cement (Fuji Plus GC Corp., Tokyo, Japan). Slight modification of the alveolar mucosa in the area of the 11 and 21 pontics allowed for the seating of the ovate tissue surface of each pontic. The retainers, replacement teeth 12 and 22, were supported by the NN implants (prosthetic diameter of 3.5 mm) and allowed for a relative narrow contour in the cervical region of each retainer crown (Figs 32 – 34). The accurate surgical placement of the implants also provided an optimal relationship between the lateral incisor replacements and the natural cuspid teeth. The relationship of the pontics to the ridge and to the retainers allowed for an acceptable interproximal soft-tissue architecture to be created.

The patient was reviewed postoperatively two weeks following delivery with no complications. At a subsequent review following a further eight weeks, the soft tissue response was excellent, and some minor adjustments of the incisal edges of the fixed dental prosthesis were made at the patient's request.

At the 2-year review, periimplant tissue health was excellent, with stable mucosal marginal tissue levels and the maintenance of good esthetics (Fig 35). Radiographic examination confirmed stable bone conditions at both implants (Figs 36 – 37).

Acknowledgments

Laboratory Procedures
John Lucas – Intra Oral Technologies, Melbourne, Australia.

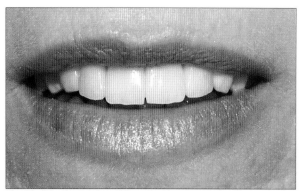

Figs 33 – 34   Frontal view of the patient in repose and smiling at the time of cementation of the FDP.

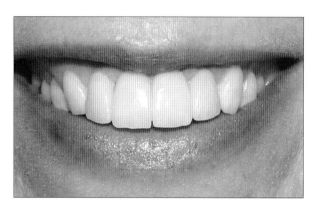

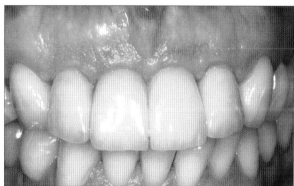

Fig 35   Frontal view of the FDP at the 2-year review. Note the stable mucosal conditions.

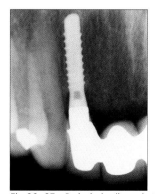
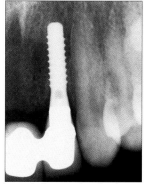

Figs 36 – 37   Periapical radiographs taken at the 2-year review, showing stable bone conditions.

4.16 Replacement of the Four Maxillary Incisors with a Fixed Dental Prosthesis Using a Conventional Loading Protocol

F. Vailati, U. Belser

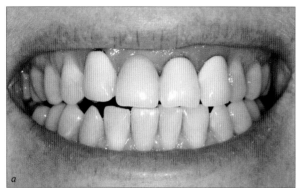

Figs 1a – b   The initial, esthetically unsatisfactory clinical situation, frontal view of the failing FDP in the anterior maxilla.

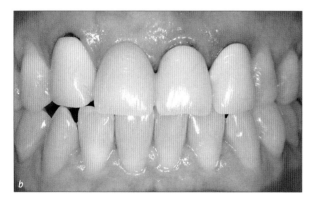

In 2005, a 54-year-old female patient presented to the University of Geneva School of Dentistry with a failing conventional fixed dental prosthesis (FDP) (Figs 1a – b). Her chief complaint was pain in the area of the premaxilla. She was a non-smoker, and her medical history was without significant findings.

Her dental history, on the other hand, showed that, earlier in life, the patient had undergone orthodontic treatment to compensate for congenitally missing maxillary lateral incisors. The two first premolars had been mesialized into the canine position, while the two canines were moved to the lateral position. Later on, when the patient lost her right central incisor, the canines served as abutment teeth for a four-unit FDP.

The patient presented a high lip line, which dramatically displayed discolored roots, an amalgam of pigmentations, and disharmonious gingival levels (Fig 2).

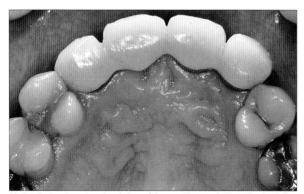

Fig 2   Pretreatment occlusal view of the maxillary arch. Note that both first premolars are in the canine position.

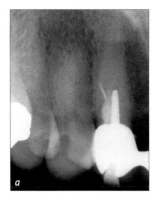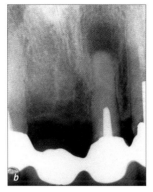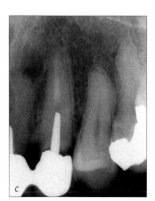

Figs 3a–c   Initial periapical radiographs showing severely compromised abutment teeth at sites 12, 21, and 22.

The radiographic and clinical examinations revealed that the three abutment teeth at sites 12, 21, and 22 were affected by recurrent caries lesions, periapical pathology, and possible root fracture (Figs 3a–c). All of them were devitalized teeth restored with rather short metal posts and crowns. The endodontic treatments and the fit of the crown margins were inadequate.

Since all three abutments were considered not restorable, they were extracted, and a provisional removable partial denture was delivered to the patient. After two months of healing, the patient was scheduled for implant placement.

At the University of Geneva, in the case of four missing maxillary incisors, the standard of care is to place two implants in the lateral position to support a four-unit FDP. Strategically, this choice avoids placing implants next to each other while maintaining the mechanical stability (Vailati and Belser, 2007).

Based on a diagnostic set-up, the ideal size of the four incisors was evaluated to guide the fabrication of the surgical template and the choice of the implant size. It was evident that only with smaller implants would the patient have a natural emergence profile both at the level of the implants and the pontics. Consequently, two Straumann Standard Plus Narrow Neck implants (endosteal diameter,

3.3 mm, length, 10 mm; Narrow Neck prosthetic platform, 3.5 mm) were placed in sites 12 and 22, following a submerged protocol. This treatment option enhances the esthetic result in patients where the lack of space in the anterior region of the maxilla may represent a restorative challenge.

The choice of a smaller implant was also justified by the occlusal scheme of the patient. Due to the minimal vertical overlap (overbite) required to re-establish function and esthetics, less detrimental lateral forces on the implant prosthesis junction were anticipated.

A conventional loading protocol (the loading of the implant after a healing period of 3 to 6 months (Ganeles and Wismeijer, 2004) was considered. The authors did not feel comfortable accelerating the loading of the two Straumann Standard Plus Narrow Neck implants because of their smaller total surface.

In the limited existing literature on immediate loading and restoration in the maxilla (Ganeles and Wismeijer, 2004), investigators generally recommended replacing multiple missing teeth with a maximum number of implants (preferably one implant for each tooth) to guarantee better initial stabilization (Degidi and Piattelli, 2003).

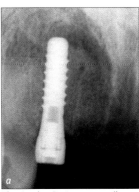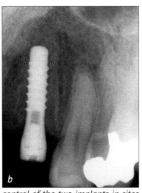

Figs 4a–b   Post-surgery radiographic control of the two implants in sites 12 and 22. The implants were placed following a submerged protocol.

However, the policy at the University of Geneva is just the opposite: this means using the minimum number of implants in the anterior quadrant to achieve the most predictable esthetic result.

In fact, in this specific case, only two implants were planned to support a four-unit FDP. No articles on early loading on reduced diameter implants supporting FDPs in the premaxilla were, or are, available. Without any literature support, a conventional loading protocol was preferred.

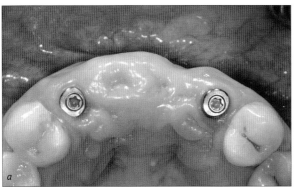

Figs 5a–c   The clinical situation after two months of osseointegration, occlusal and frontal views. At this time, a decision was made to proceed with the impression for the fabrication of a provisional FDP.

After the implant surgery, the removable prosthesis was modified at the cervical level in order not to apply any pressure on the underlying mucosa of the premaxilla.

When the patient came back after two months, second stage surgery was not necessary, since the healing caps were already exposed (Figs 5a – b). Instead, it was decided to take an impression for the fabrication of a provisional FDP. As illustrated in Fig 5, the mucosa at the level of the premaxilla was not ready to receive the final prosthesis. The conditioning of the soft tissue with a provisional restoration is a fundamental step to help the dental technician achieve a natural emergence profile with the final FDP.

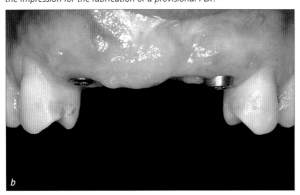

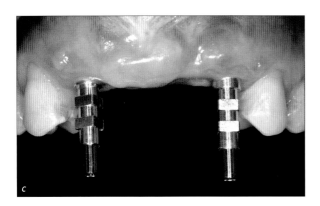

Generally, the shape of the pontics for a provisional FDP is arbitrarily carved on the cast by the dental technician. However, in this specific patient, the mucosa between the two implants appeared hypertrophic. Since there was a suspicion that some of the bone graft material was present underneath, interfering with the mucosa conditioning, a bone mapping of the premaxilla was performed.

With the information about the level of thickness of the underlying mucosa, the dentist carved the final form of the two ovate pontics (teeth 11 and 21) on the cast and returned it to the laboratory technician for the fabrication of the provisional restoration.

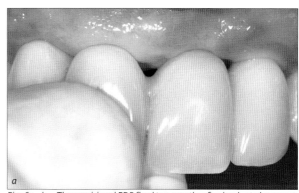

Figs 6a – b   The provisional FDP, fixed two months after implant placement. A conventional loading protocol was used. Slight blanching of the mucosa indicated the start of the soft-tissue conditioning process.

On the day of delivery of the provisional FDP (3 months after implant surgery), the degree of soft-tissue compression was clinically evaluated. Sometimes several sessions are necessary in order to obtain the esthetically pleasing emergence profile of the pontics and to avoid the risk of possible necrosis following excessive compression (Figs 6a – b).

In this patient, the soft-tissue conditioning was performed in three visits over the course of 2 months, by adding and reshaping the contour of the two pontics.

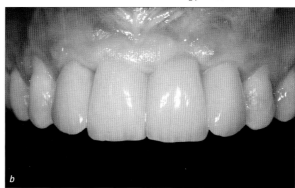

The reduced diameter of the Straumann Standard Plus Narrow Neck implants (3.5 mm shoulder diameter versus the 4.8 mm diameter of implants with Regular Neck prosthetic platform) allowed for the immediate creation of pleasing and harmonious emergence profiles at sites 12 and 22.

The provisional prosthesis was immediately placed in full occlusion. Specifically, with the prosthesis in place, the patient demonstrated group function bilaterally, while in protrusion the load was distributed mainly on the two central incisors (conventional loading protocol). However, thanks to the patient's minimal horizontal overlap (2 mm at the level of the two central incisors), less mechanical load was expected on the provisional FDP (shallow anterior guidance).

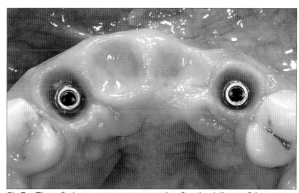

Fig 7   The soft-tissue contours two months after the delivery of the conventionally loaded provisional FDP prior to impression taking, occlusal view.

The provisional FDP was screw-retained, and it was tightened to the implants by hand.

It remained in situ for two months to create stable, esthetically pleasing soft-tissue contours (Fig 7).

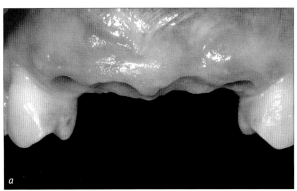

Once the emergence profile of the restoration was considered satisfactory, an impression was made for the fabrication of the final screw-retained metal-ceramic prosthesis, (Figs 8a – b), and its high-noble metal framework was cast.

The transocclusally screw-retained framework was tried in the patient's mouth in order to ensure passive fit on the implants. A radiographic control confirmed the optimal adaptation to the implant shoulders. Furthermore, the framework outline was controlled to optimally support the veneering ceramic for strength and esthetics (Figs 9a – b).

Figs 8a – b   An open-tray impression was taken to capture the mucosa conditioning and fabricate the final FDP.

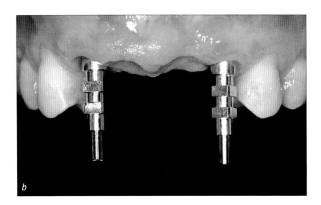

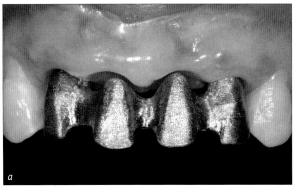

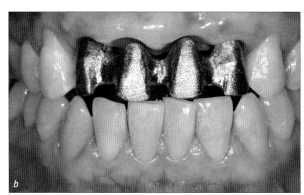

Figs 9a – b   At the metal try-in, the shape, dimension, and fit of the framework were meticulously checked and adapted.

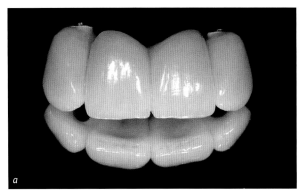

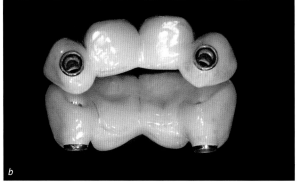

Figs 10a – b   The implant-supported, transocclusally screw-retained ceramo-metal four-unit final FDP before delivery, labial and palatal aspects. To compensate for the slight interproximal soft-tissue deficiencies, long interproximal contact lines were established to support the interdental papillae and to prevent "black interproximal triangles."

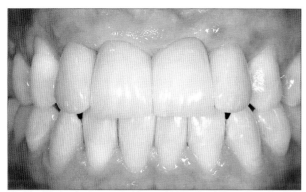

Fig 11   The implant-supported four-unit FDP after delivery. Note the slight blanching of the mucosa caused by the applied compression. After a short time, the blanching had already disappeared.

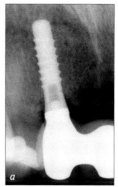
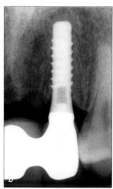

Figs 12a – b   Periapical radiographs after the delivery of the transocclusally screw-retained four-unit FDP four months after implant placement.

The same occlusal scheme adopted and tested with the provisional FDP was used for the final FDP. In the lateral movements, the patient presented group function due to the relationship of the maxillary first premolars and the mandibular canines, which did not allow for canine guidance. In the protrusive movement, the two central incisors guided the posterior disclusion.

Following the manufacturing recommendations, the prosthesis was connected to the implants by torquing the occlusal screws to 35 Ncm. During the recall appointments (every six months), the tightness of the occlusal screws was tested. Both the screws remained tightened to 35 Ncm.

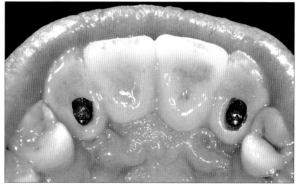

Fig 13   The palatal aspect of the final FDP on the Straumann Standard Plus Narrow Neck implants in sites 12 and 22 before the closing of the screw-access holes with composite material.

The periapical radiographs, taken after the delivery of the FDP, confirmed stable peri-implant bone conditions and precise marginal fit (Figs 12a – b).

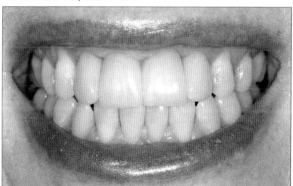

Fig 14   The smile of the patient on the day of the delivery of the implant-supported four-unit FDP.

Three-year follow-up

Clinical evidence indicates that the majority of fractures of dental prostheses occur after a period of several years. Such failures generally are not related to an episode of acute overload, but result from fatigue (high numbers of relatively low loads). There are reasonable concerns when subjecting Narrow Neck implants to higher occlusal loads (e.g. to support a FDP). Presently, few in-vitro studies of the mechanical performance under fatigue loading of reduced-diameter implants are available (Andersen and coworkers, 2001; Berglundh and coworkers, 2002; Çehreli and Akca, 2004; Comfort and coworkers, 2005; Hallmann, 2001; Romeo and coworkers, 2006; Wiskott and coworkers, 2004; Zarone and coworkers, 2006; Zinsli and coworkers, 2004). Clinically, the complication rate that should be expected when using Narrow Neck implants to support multiple-unit FDPs over an observation period of at least five years, still needs to be determined.

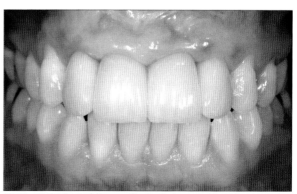

Fig 15   At the 3-year follow up after implant surgery, the FDP supported by two NN implants is nicely integrated in the patient's mouth.

Consequently, at the University of Geneva all the patients restored using NN implants to support FDP's are subject to a strict recall schedule.

At the 3-year follow-up of this specific case, the FDP was still functioning with a high level of patient satisfaction.

This case report has described the treatment planning and execution of an implant-supported FDP in a patient with four missing maxillary incisors. The implant choice, two Straumann Standard Plus Narrow Neck implants in a lateral position to support a four-unit FDP, guaranteed the most predictable esthetic result.

Due to a lack of evidence in the literature regarding the clinical performance of similar cases, the most conservative loading protocol was preferred. The implants were allowed to heal for 3 months before a provisional FDP was delivered and placed in full occlusion. The final prosthesis, reproducing the features of the provisional FDP, was then delivered 6 months after the implant surgery.

Acknowledgments

Prosthodontic Support
Dr. Giovanna Vaglio – DMD, University of Geneva, Switzerland.

Laboratory Procedures
Dominique Vinci – Master Dental Technician, University of Geneva, Switzerland.

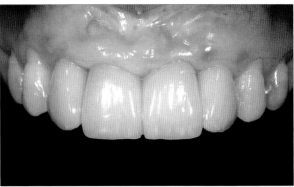

Fig 16   Close-up view of the prosthesis. Note the soft-tissue stability around the pontics. Unfortunately, the esthetic result is compromised by the presence of the preexisting amalgam tattoos. The patient, however, was indifferent to their presence.

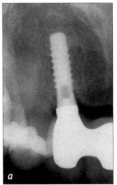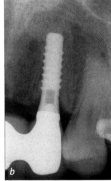

Figs 17a – b   Periapical radiograph of the two NN implants in positions 12 and 22, 3 years after the insertion.

5 Conclusions Regarding Loading Decisions for the Partially Dentate Maxilla or Mandible

D. Morton, D. Buser

5.1 Introduction

There are many factors that influence the selection of appropriate loading protocols for partially dentate patients. The relative importance of these factors varies depending on the arch, whether the restoration is in the anterior or posterior region of the mouth, and the goals of therapy.

While implant survival and treatment success is considered well-documented for partially dentate patients, the body of scientific evidence supporting varying loading protocols is inconsistent. Conventional and early loading protocols for modern root-form, screw-type implants characterized by micro-rough surfaces are both well-documented and equally predictable with regard to treatment outcome. While immediate loading in partially dentate situations is possible, the body of existing evidence is less extensive, and as such, these procedures cannot yet be recommended with the same degree of confidence.

Treatment of this type should therefore be reserved for skilled and experienced clinicians or teams, with a thorough knowledge of possible risks and complications.

Conventional loading protocols (>3 months of undisturbed healing) may provide an advantage over early loading only in specific circumstances, including poor bone density (type 4 and/or grafted bone) or quantity. Conventional loading should also be considered when general health and healing is compromised. Such conditions may include controlled diabetes or steroid or bisphosphonate therapy. In the absence of such conditions, however, conventional loading protocols are associated with unnecessary delays in treatment and are therefore less beneficial than early loading protocols, which in most circumstances should be therefore considered routine.

5.2 Degree of Treatment Difficulty

The degree of treatment difficulty for implant patients was addressed in a consensus meeting of the International Team for Implantology in early 2007. For a range of clinical indications, treatment can be classified as straightforward, advanced, or complex (A. Dawson and S. Chen, The SAC Classification in Implant Dentistry, ITI SAC Consensus Conference 2007, in preparation).

The majority of patients who require the restoration of distal extension situations or single missing teeth in the posterior maxilla or mandible fall into the straightforward treatment category (Table 1).

Table 1   Treatment Difficulty: Posterior Extended Edentulous Spaces.

Posterior extended edentulous spaces	Notes	Straightforward	Advanced	Complex
Esthetic risk	Refer to ITI Treatment Guide 1 for Esthetic Risk Assessment	Low	Moderate or high	
Access		Good	Restricted	Poor access prevents implant therapy
Interarch distance	Refers to the distance from the proposed implant's restorative margin to the opposing occlusion	> 8 mm	≤ 8 mm or > 16 mm	
Mesiodistal space		From the anatomic space corresponding to the missing teeth ± 1 mm	From the anatomic space corresponding missing teeth varies by > 1 mm	Non-restorable without adjunctive preparatory therapy due to severe space discrepancy
Occlusion/ articulation		Harmonious	Irregular but with no need for correction	Changes to existing occlusion necessary
Provisional restorations during healing		None needed	Removable or fixed	
Occlusal parafunction	Risk of complication to the restoration is high	Absent		Present
Loading protocol	To date, immediate restoration and loading procedures lack long-term scientific documentation	Conventional or early	Immediate	
Cemented (Consensus Statement)		Accessible restorative margin	Sub-mucosal location of restorative margin	
Screw-retained		Multiple non-splinted implants	Multiple splinted implants	

D. Morton, D. Buser

By selecting conventional or early loading protocols, clinicians can anticipate, for most patients, a reduced likelihood of complications during treatment and a positive outcome (Figs 1 – 4).

The replacement of single missing posterior teeth is, for the most part, also a straightforward therapy (Table 2). Inexperienced clinicians, with appropriate implant-related education, should be encouraged to treat patients exhibiting distal extension situations and single missing posterior teeth, provided additional risk factors are not evident or are well-controlled. Access to more experienced mentors should be available as necessary.

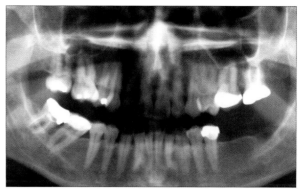

Fig 1   Pre-treatment radiograph illustrating the distal extension situation.

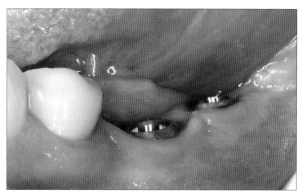

Fig 2   Healed implants six weeks subsequent to placement.

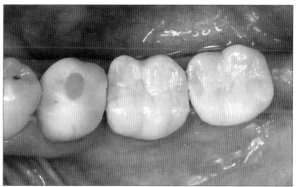

Fig 3   Definitive crowns 12 months subsequent to delivery.

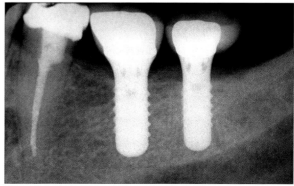

Fig 4   Periapical radiograph 12 months after loading.

Table 2   Treatment Difficulty: Posterior Single Missing Teeth.

Posterior single tooth	Notes	Straightforward	Advanced	Complex
Inter-arch distance	Refers to the distance from the proposed implant's restorative margin to the opposing occlusion	Ideal tooth height up to ± 2 mm	Reduced tooth height ≥ 2 mm	Non-restorable without adjunctive preparatory therapy, due to severe overeruption of the opposing dentition
Mesiodistal space (premolar)		Anatomic space corresponding to the missing tooth ± 1 mm	Anatomic space corresponding to the missing tooth plus 2 mm or more	Non-restorable without adjunctive preparatory therapy, due to severe space restriction (≤ 5 mm)
Mesiodistal space (molar)		Anatomic space corresponding to the missing tooth ± 1 mm	Anatomic space corresponding to the missing tooth ± 2 mm or more	Non-restorable without adjunctive preparatory therapy, due to severe space restriction (≤ 5 mm)
Access		Adequate	Restricted	Access prohibits implant therapy
Loading protocol	To date, immediate restoration and loading procedures lack long-term scientific documentation	Conventional or early	Immediate	
Esthetic risk	Refer to ITI Treatment Guide 1 for Esthetic Risk Assessment	Low	Moderate	Maxillary first premolars in with high esthetic demands
Occlusal parafuntion	Risk of complication to the restoration is high	Absent		Present
Provisional implant-supported restorations	Provisional restorations are recommended	Restorative margin ≤ 3 mm apical to mucosal crest	Restorative margin > 3 mm apical to mucosal crest	

Immediate loading protocols for distal extension situations and posterior single missing teeth are associated with additional, technique-sensitive clinical procedures. As such, this treatment should be considered advanced. The benefit of reduced treatment time for patients receiving immediate loading for these indications should be carefully and accurately assessed against the increased risk of complication, particularly early implant loss. Occlusal loads in the posterior areas of the mouth are much greater than those in the anterior, and protection from these forces, particularly for distal extension situations, is more difficult to obtain and manage. For this reason, restorative dentists and their surgical colleagues should have more experience and they should display a greater degree of comfort with the more difficult procedures.

The replacement of single missing teeth in the anterior maxilla is made more difficult by the need for an esthetic outcome. This increases the importance of a team approach to the planning and delivery of the treatment. Pre-treatment esthetic risk assessment should be mandatory for these patients, with emphasis placed on evaluating the patient's esthetic expectations, lip line, tissue biotype, periodontal and restorative condition (particularly of adjacent teeth), tooth shape, and edentulous span. Increasing the assessment and planning requirements categorizes the surgical and restorative treatment as advanced, and on rare occasions even as complex (Table 3).

Table 3   *Treatment Difficulty: Anterior Single Missing Teeth.*

Anterior single tooth	Notes	Straightforward	Advanced	Complex
Intermaxillary relationship	Refers to horizontal and vertical overlap and the effect on restorability and esthetic outcome	Class I and III	Class II Div 1 and 2	Non-restorable without adjunctive preparatory therapy, due to severe malocclusion
Mesiodistal space (maxillary central)	Symmetry is essential for a successful outcome		Symmetry ± 1 mm of contra-lateral tooth	Asymmetry greater than 1 mm
Mesiodistal space (maxillary laterals and canines)		Symmetry ± 1 mm of contra-lateral tooth	Asymmetry greater than 1 mm	
Mesiodistal space (mandibular anterior)		Symmetry ± 1 mm of contra-lateral tooth	Asymmetry greater than 1 mm	
Loading protocol	To date, immediate restoration and loading procedures lack long-term scientific documentation		Conventional or early	Immediate
Esthetic risk	Refer to ITI Treatment Guide 1 for Esthetic Risk Assessment		Low or moderate	High
Occlusal parafuntion	Risk of complication to the restoration not implant survival	Absent		Present
Provisional implant-supported restorations	Provisional restorations are highly recommended or mandatory		Restorative margin ≤ 3 mm apical to mucosal crest	Restorative margin > 3 mm apical to mucosal crest

For patients receiving implants in the anterior maxilla, there is a greater demand on accurate three-dimensional, restoration-driven implant placement, often in conjunction with hard and soft tissue augmentation procedures (Figs 5 – 10).

The replacement of adjacent missing teeth in the anterior maxilla presents a far greater challenge (Table 4). The response of the supporting hard and soft tissues to the implant position and restorative method is unpredictable, and the risk to the esthetic outcome is magnified. As most patients in this category are interested primarily in a pleasing esthetic outcome, the esthetic risk is almost always increased; these cases should be considered complex, irrespective of the loading methodology. Clinicians should be mindful of misinformation associated with loading protocols, particularly immediate loading, for patients with extended edentulous spaces in the esthetic zone. Treatment should be reserved for the most skilled and experienced clinicians or teams.

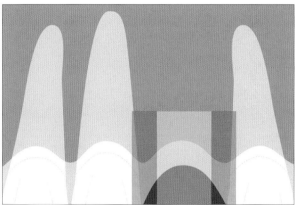

Fig 5 Correct implant position in the mesiodistal comfort zone (green).

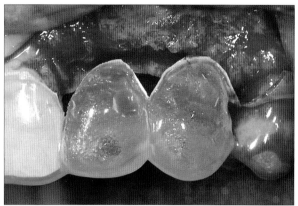

Fig 8 Depth guide used to confirm appropriate depth of implant subsequent to placement.

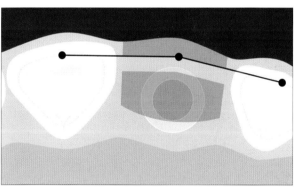

Fig 6 Orofacial comfort (green) and danger zones (red).

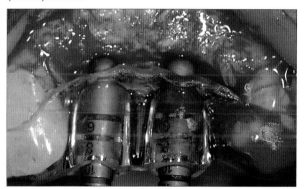

Fig 9 Surgical template communicating desired mesio-distal and oro-facial implant position.

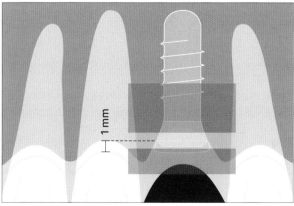

Fig 7 Comfort (green) and danger zones (red) in the coronoapical dimension.

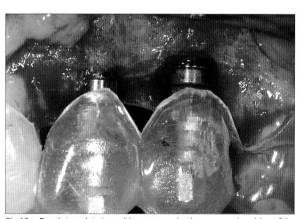

Fig 10 Depth template in position communicating proposed position of the final mucosal margin.

Table 4   Treatment Difficulty: Anterior Extended Edentulous Spaces.

Anterior extended edentulous spaces	Notes	Straightforward	Advanced	Complex
Esthetic risk	Refer to ITI Treatment Guide 1 for Esthetic Risk Assessment		Low or moderate	High
Intermaxillary relationship	Refers to the horizontal and vertical overlap and the effect on restorability and esthetic outcome		Class I and III Class II Div 1 and 2	Non-restorable without adjunctive preparatory therapy, due to severe malocclusion
Mesiodistal space			Adequate for required tooth replacement Insufficient space available for the replacement of the missing teeth	Adjunctive therapy necessary to replace all missing teeth
Occlusion/articulation			Harmonious Irregular with no need for correction	Changes to existing occlusion necessary
Provisional restorations during healing			Removable Fixed	
Provisional implant-supported restorations	Provisional restorations are highly recommended or mandatory		Restorative margin ≤ 3 mm apical to mucosal crest	Restorative margin > 3 mm apical to mucosal crest
Occlusal parafuntion	Risk of complication to the restoration not implant survival	Absent		Present
Loading protocol	To date, immediate restoration and loading procedures lack long-term scientific documentation			Conventional or early Immediate

Additional factors influence the treatment difficulty associated with all loading protocols for particular regional indications. It is relatively common to encounter limitations in interocclusal space or occlusal plane disharmony in distal-extension and posterior edentulous situations, particularly when oligodontia or posterior edentulism has gone untreated for a long time (Fig 11).

These difficulties can be the result of limited oral opening and overeruption or the drifting of the opposing or adjacent teeth. Such restrictions can complicate or prevent both the surgical placement and the restoration of implants by restricting access. For single missing teeth in the posterior areas of the mouth, the drifting of adjacent teeth can negatively affect the mesiodistal distance available for implant placement and restoration, and poor adjacent tooth inclination can lead to maintenance difficulties. A careful evaluation of these factors will on occasion indicate the need for adjunctive orthodontic treatment prior to implant therapy (Fig 12).

For these patients, the risk to the treatment outcome can increase as a result of the additional procedures and the need for occlusal modifications. This is particularly relevant in patients exhibiting bruxism, where treatment is considered complex. For single and multiple missing teeth in the anterior maxilla, symmetry and tooth inclination can also be indications for orthodontic therapy prior to implant treatment (Fig 13). Space limitations can result from horizontal and vertical overlap associated with crowding and malocclusions. These conditions are more likely to be associated with compromised treatment outcomes.

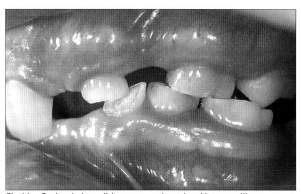

Fig 11   Occlusal plane disharmony and restricted intermaxillary space resulting from oligodontia and the long-term retention of deciduous teeth.

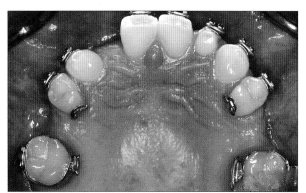

Fig 12   Orthodontic therapy to improve tooth alignment and optimize symmetry and space dimensions in edentulous areas.

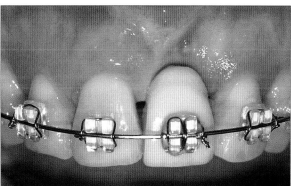

Fig 13   Orthodontic therapy to improve space symmetry and the long-axis inclination of adjacent teeth.

The character of the local anatomy should be considered when choosing a loading protocol. The quality and quantity of bone, particularly in the posterior maxilla and mandible, should be carefully evaluated in conjunction with the surgical team members. The need for supplemental surgical procedures (to avoid the maxillary sinus and inferior alveolar canal and contents) may increase the risk to the treatment outcome when accelerated loading is utilized.

Restorative procedures for distal extension situations and single missing posterior teeth are, for the most part, not difficult. Cemented restorations are recommended, using either solid or two-piece cementable abutments. Impression procedures are not challenging and do not involve customized procedures. While provisional restorations are recommended, they are not considered mandatory for these patients, as the esthetic maturation of the soft tissues is often not necessary for a successful outcome. The restorative procedures for these treatment indications are therefore considered straightforward.

Restoring implants in the anterior maxilla is more demanding. Often, the restorative margin is positioned 2 – 5 millimeters below the mucosa, especially on the approximal aspects. Screw-retained prostheses at implant level are recommended in these cases. This increases the degree of treatment difficulty for both the clinician and the laboratory technician. Provisional restorations are mandatory in order to shape and mature the soft tissue surrounding the restoration and to maximize esthetic predictability. For these reasons, the restoration of single teeth in the esthetic zone is considered advanced, and adjacent missing teeth are considered complex.

There is no question that patients benefit from reduced time to loading. An earlier placement of provisional and definitive restorations establishes occlusion and esthetics sooner, thus improving masticatory function, comfort, and psychological satisfaction. For all partially dentate situations, it has been established that early loading (6 – 8 weeks of undisturbed healing) of implants with a microroughened surface can accomplish these goals with no reduction in predictability or increase in risk when compared to conventional protocols. For this reason, early loading should be considered routine. The period of undisturbed healing may be further reduced with improvements in implant surface morphology or chemistry, and an enhanced biologic response to implants.

Although they maximize the advantage of reduced treatment time, immediate loading protocols for partially edentulous patients lack quality scientific support. In particular, the risk of early implant loss cannot be ignored. The transfer of occlusal load to the immature bone-implant interface has the potential to destabilize the implant and prevent osseointegration. These risks are maximized in posterior edentulous spaces, where forces are greatest, and when the implant-supported restorations cannot be protected by surrounding teeth. With excellent results observed for early loading, the limited gain in treatment time associated with immediate loading may present an unreasonable risk.

For these reasons, early loading protocols for the majority of partially dentate patients represent a cost-effective and sound treatment choice, in terms of both expense and time. Conventional loading protocols are often not effective in terms of time, and immediate loading can be associated with unnecessary risk.

5.3 Conclusions: Loading Protocols for Partially Dentate Patients

Table 5   Factors Influencing Loading Decisions for Distal Extension Situations.

Decision factor	Loading protocol		
	Conventional	Early	Immediate
Scientific documentation	Good	Good	Moderate
Treatment difficulty (SAC)	S	S	A
Benefit to patient	Reduced (time)	High	Reduced (risk)
Risk of complication	Low	Low	Moderate
Cost-effectiveness	Good	Good	Reduced

S = Straightforward, A = Advanced

Table 6   Factors influencing loading decisions for posterior single missing teeth.

Decision factor	Loading protocol		
	Conventional	Early	Immediate
Scientific documentation	Good	Good	Moderate
Treatment difficulty (SAC)	S	S	A
Benefit to patient	Reduced (time)	High	Reduced (risk)
Risk of complication	Low	Low	Moderate
Cost-effectiveness	Good	Good	Reduced

S = Straightforward, A = Advanced

Table 7   Factors Influencing Loading Decisions for Anterior Single Missing Teeth.

	Loading protocol		
	Conventional	**Early**	**Immediate**
Decision factor			
Scientific documentation	Good	Good	Low
Treatment difficulty (SAC)	A	A	C
Benefit to patient	Reduced (time)	High	Reduced (risk)
Risk of complication	Low	Low	High
Cost-effectiveness	Reduced	Reduced	Reduced

A = Advanced, C = Complex

Table 8   Factors Influencing Loading Decisions for Anterior Multiple Missing Teeth.

	Loading protocol		
	Conventional	**Early**	**Immediate**
Decision factor			
Scientific documentation	Moderate	Moderate	Low
Treatment difficulty (SAC)	C	C	C
Benefit to patient	Reduced (time)	High	Reduced (risk)
Risk of complication	Moderate	Moderate	High
Cost-effectiveness	Reduced	Reduced	Reduced

C = Complex

6 Literature/References

Abrahamsson I, Cardaropoli G. Peri-implant hard and soft tissue integration to dental implants made of titanium and gold. Clinical Oral Impl Res. 2007 Jun;18(3):269–74. Epub 2007 Feb 13.

Adell R, Lekholm U, Rockler B, Brånemark PI. A 15-year study of osseointegrated implants in the treatment of the edentulous jaw. Int J Oral Surg. 1981 Dec;10(6):387–416.

Adell R, Eriksson B, Lekholm U, Brånemark PI, Jemt T. A long-term follow-up study of osseointegrated implants in the treatment of totally edentulous jaws. Int J Oral Maxillofac Implants. 1990 Winter;5(4): 347–59.

Akagawa Y, Hashimoto M, Kondo N, Satomi K, Takata T, Tsuru H. Initial bone-implant interfaces of submergible and supramergible endosseous single-crystal sapphire implants. J Prosthet Dent. 1986 Jan;55(1):96–100.

Albrektsson T, Brånemark PI, Hansson HA, Lindström J. Osseointegrated titanium implants. Requirements for ensuring a long-lasting, direct bone-to-implant anchorage in man. Acta Orthop Scand. 1981;52(2):155–70.

Albrektsson T. Direct bone anchorage of dental implants. J Prosthet Dent. 1983 Aug;50(2):255–61.

Albrektsson T. Principles of osseointegration. In: Hobkirk JA, Watson RM, editor. Color atlas and text of dental and maxillofacial implantology. St Louis: Mosby; 1995. p. 9–19.

Amsterdam M, Abrams L. Periodontal prosthesis . In: Goldman HM, Cohen DW, editors. Periodontal Therapy. 5th ed.. St. Louis: Mosby; 1973. p. 990–993.

Andersen E, Saxegaard E, Knutsen BM, Haanaes HR. A prospective clinical study evaluating the safety and effectiveness of narrow-diameter threaded implants in the anterior region of the maxilla. Int J Oral Maxillofac Implants. 2001 Mar–Apr;16(2):217–24.

Aparicio C, Rangert B, Sennerby L. Immediate/early loading of dental implants: a report from the Sociedad Española de Implantes World Congress consensus meeting in Barcelona, Spain, 2002. Clin Implant Dent Relat Res. 2003;5(1):57–60.

Arvidson K, Bystedt H, Frykolm A, von Konow L, Lothius E. Five-year prospective follow-up report on the Astra Tech Dental Implant System in the treatment of edentulous mandibles. Clin Oral Implants Res. 1998 Aug;9(4):225–34.

Attard NJ, Zarb GA. Immediate and early implant loading protocols: a literature review of clinical studies. J Prosthet Dent. 2005 Sep;94(3):242–58.

Babbush CA. Titanium plasma spray screw implant system for reconstruction of the edentulous mandible. Dent Clin North Am. 1986 Jan;30(1):117–31.

Babbush CA, Kent JN, Misiek DJ. Titanium plasma-sprayed (TPS) screw implants for the reconstruction of the edentulous mandible. J Oral Maxillofac Surg. 1986 Apr;44(4):274–82.

Barone A, Rispoli L, Vozza I, Quaranta A, Covani U. Immediate restoration of single implants placed immediately after tooth extraction. J Periodontol. 2006 Nov;77(11):1914–20.

Becker W, Becker BE, Huffstetler S. Early functional loading at 5 days for Brånemark implants placed into edentulous mandibles: a prospective, open-ended, longitudinal study. J Periodontol. 2003 May;74(5):695–702.

Behneke A, Behneke N, d'Hoedt B. A 5-year longitudinal study of the clinical effectiveness of ITI solid-screw implants in the treatment of mandibular edentulism. Int J Oral Maxillofac Implants. 2002 Nov-Dec;17(6):799–810.

Belser UC, Schmid B, Higginbottom F, Buser D. Outcome analysis of implant restorations located in the anterior maxilla: a review of the recent literature. Int J Oral Maxillofac Implants. 2004;19 Suppl:30–42.

Berglundh T, Persson L, Klinge B. (2002) A systematic review of the incidence of biological and technical complications in implant dentistry reported in prospective longitudinal studies of at least 5 years. J Clin Periodontol. 2002;29 Suppl 3:197-212; discussion 232–3.

Bergkvist G, Sahlholm S, Nilner K, Lindh C. Implant supported fixed prostheses in the edentulous maxilla: a 2-year clinical and radiological follow-up of treatment with non-submerged ITI implants. Clin Oral Implants Res. 2004 Jun;15(3):351–9.

Brånemark PI, Zarb G, Albrektsson T. Tissue-integrated prosthesis: osseointegration in clinical dentistry. Chicago: Quintessence; 1985. p. 11 – 77.

Brånemark PI. The Brånemark Novum protocol for same-day teeth: a global perspective. Chicago: Quintessence; 2001. p. 9 – 29.

Brånemark PI, Hansson BO, Adell R, Breine U, Lindström J, Hallen O, Ohman A. Osseointegrated implants in the treatment of the edentulous jaw: experience from a 10-year period. Scand J Plast Reconstr Surg Suppl. 1977;16:1-132.

Brunski JB, Moccia AF Jr, Pollock SR, Korostoff E, Trachtenberg DI. The influence of functional use of endosseous dental implants on the tissue-implant interface: I. Histological aspects. J Dent Res. 1979 Oct;58(10):1953 – 69.

Büchter A, Kleinheinz J, Wiesmann HP, Jayaranan M, Joos U, Meyer U. Interface reaction at dental implants inserted in condensed bone. Clin Oral Implants Res. 2005 Oct;16(5):509 – 17.

Buser D, Mericske-Stern R, Bernard JP, Behneke A, Behneke N, Hirt HP, et al. Long-term evaluation of non-submerged ITI implants. Part 1: 8-year life table analysis of prospective multi-center study with 2359 implants. Clin Oral Implants Res. 1997 Jun;8(3):161 – 72.

Buser D, Martin W, Belser UC. Optimizing esthetics for implant restorations in the anterior maxilla: Anatomic and surgical considerations. Int J Oral Maxillofac Implants. 2004;19 Suppl:43 – 61.

Buser D, Belser UC, Wismeijer D, editors. ITI Treatment Guide, Vol I: Implant therapy in the esthetic zone for single-tooth replacements. Chicago: Quintessence; 2006.

Calandriello R, Tomatis M, Rangert B. Immediate functional loading of Brånemark system implants with enhanced initial stability: a prospective 1- to 2- year clinical and radiographic study. Clin Implant Dent Relat Res 2003;5(suppl 1):57 – 63.

Calandriello R, Tomatis M, Vallone R, Rangert B, Gottlow J. Immediate occlusal loading using Brånemark system wide-platform TiUnite implants: an interim report of a prospective open-ended clinical multicenter study. Clin Implant Dent Relat Res. 2003;5 Suppl 1:10 – 20.

Cameron H, Pilliar RM, Macnab I. The effect of movement on the bonding of porous metal to bone. J Biomed Mater Res. 1973 Jul;7(4):301 – 11.

Çehreli MC, Akca K. Narrow-diameter implants as terminal support for occlusal three-unit FPDs: a biomechanical analysis. Int J Periodontics Restorative Dent. 2004 Dec;24(6):513 – 9.

Chaushu G, Chaushu S, Tzohar A, Dayan D. Immediate loading of single-tooth implants: immediate versus non-immediate implantation. A clinical report. Int J Oral Maxillofac Implants. 2001 Mar-Apr;16(2):267 – 72.

Chiapasco M, Gatti C, Rossi E, Haefliger W, Markwalder T. Implant-retained mandibular overdentures with immediate loading: A retrospective multicenter study on 226 consecutive cases. Clin Oral Implants Res. 1997 Feb;8(1):48 – 57.

Chiapasco M. Early and immediate restoration and loading of implants in completely edentulous patients. Int J Oral Maxillofac Implants. 2004;19 Suppl:76 – 91.

Choquet V, Hermans M, Adriaenssens P, Daelemans P, Tarnow DP, Malevez C. Clinical and radiographic evaluation of the papilla level adjacent to single-tooth dental implants: a retrospective study in the maxillary anterior region. J Periodontol. 2001 Oct;72(10):1364 – 71.

Cochran DL. A comparison of endosseous dental implant surfaces. J Periodontol. 1999 Dec;70(12): 1523 – 39.

Cochran D, Buser D, Ten Bruggenkate CM, Weingart D, Taylor T, Bernard J, et al. The use of reduced healing times on ITI implants with a sandblasted and acid-etched (SLA) surface: early results from clinical trials on ITI SLA implants. Clin Oral Implants Res. 2002 Apr;13(2):144 – 53.

Cochran D, Morton D, Weber HP. Consensus statement and recommended clinical procedures regarding loading protocols for endosseous dental implants. Int J Oral Maxillofac Implants. 2004;19 Suppl:109 – 13.

Cochran D, Oates T, Morton D, Jones A, Buser D, Peters F. Clinical field trial examining an implant with a sandblasted and acid etch surface. J Periodontol. 2007 [submitted].

Comfort MB, Chu FC, Chai J, Wat PY, Chow TW. A 5-year prospective study on small diameter screw-shaped oral implants. J Oral Rehabil. 2005 May; 32(5): 341–5.

Cooper L, Felton DA, Kugelberg CF, Ellner S, Chaffee N, Molina AL, Moriarty JD, Paquette D, Palmqvist U. A multicenter 12-month evaluation of single-tooth implants restored 3 weeks after 1-stage surgery. Int J Oral Maxillofac Implants. 2001 Mar-Apr;16(2):182–92.

Cooper LF, Rahman A, Moriarty J, Chaffee N, Sacco D. Immediate mandibular rehabilitation with endosseous implants: simultaneous extraction, implant placement and loading. Int J Oral Maxillofac Implants. 2002 Jul-Aug;17(4):517–25.

Dawson AS, Chen S: The SAC classification in implant dentistry. ITI SAC Consensus Conference 2007 [in preparation].

Del Fabbro M, Testori T, Francetti L, Taschieri S, Weinstein R. Systematic review of survival rates for immediately loaded dental implants. Int J Periodontics Restorative Dent. 2006 Jun;26(3):249–63.

Degidi M, Piattelli A. Immediate functional and non-functional loading of dental implants: a 2- to 60-month follow-up study of 646 titanium implants. J Periodontol. 2003 Feb;74(2):225–41.

Degidi M, Gehrke P, Spanel A, Piatelli A. Syncrystallization: a technique for temporization of immediately loaded implants with metal-reinforced acrylic resin restorations. Clin Implant Dent Relat Res. 2006;8(3):123–34.

Deporter DA, Watson PA, Pilliar RM, Melcher AH, Winslow J, Howley TP, et al. A histological assessment of the initial healing response adjacent to porous-surfaced titanium alloy dental implants in dogs. Dent Res. 1986 Aug;65(8):1064–70.

Ekfeldt A, Christiansson U, Eriksson T, Linden U, Lundqvist S, Rundcrantz T, et al. A retrospective analysis of factors associated with multiple implant failures in maxillae. Clin Oral Implants Res. 2001 Oct;12(5):462–7.

Ericsson I, Randow K, Nilner K, Peterson A. Early functional loading of Brånemark dental implants: 5-year clinical follow-up study. Clin Implant Dent Relat Res. 2000;2(2):70–7.

Ericsson I, Nilson H, Nilner K, Randow K. Immediate functional loading of Brånemark single tooth implants: An 18 months' clinical pilot follow-up study. Clin Oral Implants Res. 2000 Feb;11(1):26–33.

Ferrigno N, Laureti M, Fanali S, Grippaudo G. A long-term folllow-up of non-submered ITI implants in the treatment of totally edentulous jaws. Part I: Ten-year life table analysis of a prospective multicenter study with 1286 implants. Clin Oral Implants Res. 2002 Jun;13(3):260–73.

Fischer K, Stenberg T. Early loading of ITI implants supporting a maxillary full-arch prosthesis: 1-year data of a prospective, randomized study. Int J Oral Maxillofac Implants. 2004 May-Jun;19(3):374–81.

Fischer K, Stenberg T. Three-year data from a randomized, controlled study of early loading of single-stage dental implants supporting maxillary full-arch prostheses. Int J Oral Maxillofac Implants. 2006 Mar-Apr;21(2):245–52.

Fugazzotto PA, Vlassis J, Butler B. ITI Implant use in private practice: Clinical results with 5526 implants followed up to 72+ months in function. Int J Oral Maxillofac Implants. 2004 May-Jun;19(3):408–12.

Gallucci GO, Bernard JP, Bertosa M, Belser UC. Immediate loading with fixed screw-retained provisional restorations in edentulous jaws: the pickup technique. Int J Oral Maxillofac Implants. 2004 Jul-Aug;19(4):524–33.

Ganeles J, Wismeijer D: Early and immediately restored and loaded dental implants for single-tooth and partial-arch applications. Int J Oral Maxillofac Implants. 2004;19 Suppl:92–102.

Ganeles J, Rosenberg MM, Holt RL, Reichman LH. Immediate loading of implants with fixed restorations in the completely edentulous mandible: report of 27 patients from a private practice. Int J Oral Maxillofac Implants. 2001 May-Jun;16(3):418–26.

Gapski R, Wang HL, Mascarenhas P, Lang NP. Critical review of immediate implant loading. Clin Oral Implants Res. 2003 Oct;14(5):515–27.

Glauser R, Lundgren AK, Gottlow J, Sennerby L, Portmann M, Ruhstaller P, et al. Immediate occlusal loading of Brånemark TiUnite implants placed predominantly in soft bone: 1-year results of a prospective clinical study. Clin Implant Dent Relat Res. 2003;5 Suppl 1:47–56.

Gotfredsen K, Karlsson U. A prospective 5-year study of fixed partial prostheses supported by implant with machined and TiO$_2$-blasted surface. J Prosthodont. 2001 Mar;10(1):2 – 7.

Grunder U. Stability of the mucosal topography around single-tooth implants and adjacent teeth: 1-year results. Int J Periodontics Restorative Dent. 2000 Feb;20(1):11 – 7.

Grunder U, Gracis S, Capelli M. Influence of the 3-D bone-to-implant relationship on esthetics. Int J Periodontics Restorative Dent. 2005 Apr;25(2):113 – 9.

Haas R, Polak C, Fürhauser R, Mailath-Pokorny G, Dörtbudak O, Watzek G. A long-term follow-up of 76 Brånemark single-tooth implants. Clin Oral Implants Res. 2002 Feb;13(1):38 – 43.

Hallman M. A prospective study of treatment of severely resorbed maxillae with narrow nonsubmerged implants: results after 1 year of loading. Int J Oral Maxillofac Impl. 2001 Sep – Oct;16(5):731 – 6.

Hämmerle CH, Chen S, Wilson TG: Consensus statements and recommended clinical procedrues regarding the placement of implants in extraction sockets. Int J Oral Maxillofac Implants. 2004;19 Suppl:26 – 8.

Herrmann I, Lekholm U, Holm S, Kultje C. Evaluation of patient and implant characteristics as potential prognostic factors for oral implant failures. Int J Oral Maxillofac Implants. 2005 Mar-Apr;20(2):220 – 30.

Higginbottom FL, Wilson, TG. Three-dimensional templates for placement of root-form dental implants: a technical note. Int J Oral Maxillofac Implants. 1996 Nov-Dec;11(6):787 – 93.

Horiuchi K, Uchida H, Yamamoto K, Sugimura M. Immediate loading of Brånemark system implants following placement in edentulous patients: a clinical report. Int J Oral Maxillofac Implants. 2000 Nov-Dec;15(6):824-30.

Hui E, Chow J, Li D, Liu J, Wat P, Law H. Immediate provisional for single-tooth implant replacement with Brånemark system: preliminary report. Clin Implant Dent Relat Res. 2001;3(2):79 – 86.

Ibañez JC, Tahhan MJ, Zamar JA, Menendez AB, Juaneda AM, Zamar NJ, et al. Immediate occlusal loading of double acid-etched surface titanium implants in 41 consecutive full-arch cases in the mandible and maxilla: 6- to 74-month results. J Periodontol. 2005 Nov;76(11):1972 – 81.

Ioannidou E. Doufexi A. Does loading time affect implant survival? A meta-analysis of 1266 implants. J Periodontol. 2005 Aug;76(8):1252 – 8.

Jaffin RA, Berman CL. The excessive loss of Brånemark fixtures in type IV bone: a 5-year analysis. J Periodontol. 1991 Jan;62(1):2 – 4.

Jaffin RA, Kumar A, Berman CL. Immediate loading of dental implants in the completely edentulous maxilla: a clinical report. Int J Oral Maxillofac Implants. 2004 Sep-Oct;19(5):721 – 30.

Jemt T, Chai J, Harnett J, Heath MR, Hutton JE, Johns RB, et al. A 5-year prospective multicenter follow-up report on overdentures supported by osseointegrated implants. Int J Oral Maxillofac Implants. 1996 May-Jun;11(3):291 – 8.

Jemt T, Häger P. Early complete failures of fixed implant supported prostheses in the edentulous maxilla: a 3-year analusis of 17 consecutive cluster failure patients. Clin Implant Dent Relat Res. 2006;8(2):77 – 86.

Jokstad A, Carr A. What is the effect on outcomes of time-to-loading of a fixed or removable prosthesis placed on implant(s)? Review for the Academy of Osseointegration State of the Science of Implant Dentistry Conference 2006. Int J Oral Maxillofac Implants [accepted for publication].

Jungner M, Lundqvist P, Lundgren S. Oxidized titanium implants (Nobel Biocare TiUnite) compared with turned titanium implants (Nobel Biocare mark III) with respect to implant failure in a group of consecutive patients treated with early functional loading and two-stage protocol. Clin Oral Implants Res. 2005 Jun;16(3):308 – 12.

Juodzbalys G, Wang HL. Soft and hard tissue assessment of immediate implant placement: a case series. Clin Oral Implants Res. 2007 Apr;18(2):237 – 43.

Kan JY, Rungcharassaeng K, Lozada J. Immediate placement and provisionalization of maxillary anterior single implants: 1-year prospective study. Int J Oral Maxillofac Implants. 2003 Jan-Feb;18(1):31 – 9.

Khang W, Feldman S, Hawley CE, Gunsolley J. A multi-centered study comparing dual acid-etched and machined surface implants in various bone qualities. J Periodontol. 2001 Oct;72(10):1384-90.

Kohal RJ, Klaus G, Strub JR. Zirconia-implant-supported all-ceramic crowns withstand long-term load: a pilot investigation. Clin Oral Implants Res. 2006 Oct;17(5):565 – 71.

Lekholm U, Zarb GA. Patient selection and preparation. In: Brånemark PI, Zarb GA, Albrektsson T, editors. Tissue-integrated prostheses. osseointegration in clinical dentistry. Chicago: Quintessence; 1985. p. 199 – 209.

Lekholm U, Gunne J, Henry P, Higuchi K, Lindén U, Bergström C, et al. Survival of the Brånemark implant in partially edentulous jaws: a 10-year prospective multicenter study. Int J Oral Maxillofac Implants. 1999 Sep-Oct;14(5):639 – 45.

Levine R, Rose L, Salama H. Immediate loading of root-form implants: two case reports 3 years after loading. Int J Periodontics Restorative Dent. 1998 Aug;18(4):333 – 43.

Levine RA, Clem DS 3rd, Wilson TG Jr, Higginbottom F, Solnit G. Multicenter retrospective analysis of the ITI implant system used for single-tooth replacements: results of loading for 2 or more years. Int J Oral Maxillofac Implants. 1999 Jul-Aug;14(4):516 – 20.

Levine RA, Clem D, Beagle J, Ganeles J, Johnson P, Solnit G, et al. Multicenter retrospective analysis of the solid-screw ITI implant for posterior single-tooth replacements. Int J Oral Maxillofac Implants. 2002 Jul-Aug;17(4):550 – 6.

Levin L, Sadet P, Grossmann Y. A retrospective evaluation of 1387 single-tooth implants: a 6-year follow up. J Periodontol. 2006 Dec;77(12):2080 – 3. (2006a)

Levin L, Laviv A, Schwartz-Arad D. Long-term success of implants replacing a single molar. J Periodontol. 2006 Sep;77(9):1528 – 32. (2006b)

Lindh T, Gunne J, Tillberg A, Molin M. A meta-analysis of implants in partial edentulism. Clin Oral Implants Res. 1998 Apr;9(2):80 – 90.

Linkow LI, Glassman PE, Asnis ST. Macroscopic and microscopic studies of endosteal blade-vent implants (six-month dog study). Oral Implantol. 1973 Spring;3(4):281 – 309.

Lioubavina-Hack N, Lang NP, Karring T. Significance of primary stability for osseointegration of dental implants. Clin Oral Implants Res. 2006 Jun;17(3):244 – 50.

Misch CE, Hahn J, Judy KW, Lemons JE, Linkow LI, Lozada JL, et al. Workshop guidelines on immediate loading in implant dentistry. November 7, 2003. J Oral Implantol. 2004;30(5):283 – 8.

Molly L. Bone density and primary stability in implant therapy. Clin Oral Implants Res. 2006 Oct;17 Suppl 2:124 – 35.

Morton D, Jaffin R, Weber HP. Immediate restoration and loading of dental implants: clinical considerations and protocols. Int J Oral Maxillofac Implants. 2004;19 Suppl:103 – 8.

Naert I, Koutsikakis G, Duyck J, Quirynen M, Jacobs R, van Steenberghe D. Biologic outcome of implant-supported restorations in the treatment of partial edentulism. Part I: a longitudinal clinical evaluation. Clin Oral Implants Res. 2002 Aug;13(4):381 – 9.

Nkenke E, Lehner B, Fenner, M, Roman FS, Thams U, Neukam FW, et al. Immediate versus delayed loading of dental implants in the maxillae of minipigs: follow-up of implant stability and implant failures. Int J Oral Maxillofac Implants. 2005 Jan-Feb;20(1):39 – 47.

Nkenke E, Fenner M. Indications for immediate loading of implants and implant success. Clin Oral Implants Res. 2006 Oct;17 Suppl 2:19 – 34.

Nordin T, Nilsson R, Frykholm A, Hallman M. A 3-arm study of early loading of rough-surfaced implants in the completely edentulous maxilla and in the edentulous posterior maxilla and mandible: results after 1 year of loading. Int J Oral Maxillofac Implants. 2004 Nov-Dec;19(6):880 – 6.

Ostman PO, Hellman M, Sennerby L. Direct implant loading in the edentulous maxilla using a bone density-adapted surgical protocol and primary implant stability criteria for inclusion. Clin Implant Dent Relat Res. 2005;7 Suppl 1:S60 – 9.

Payne AG, Tawse-Smith A, Duncan WD, Kumara R. Conventional and early loading of unsplinted ITI implants supporting mandibular overdentures. Clin Oral Implants Res. 2002 Dec;13(6):603 – 9.

Priest G. Predictability of soft tissue form around single-tooth implant restorations. Int J Periodontics Restorative Dent. 2003 Feb;23(1):19 – 27.

Quirynen M, Van Assche N, Botticelli D, Berglundh T. How does the timing of Implant Placement to Extraction Affect Outcome?. Int J Oral Maxillofac Implants. 2007;22 Suppl:203 – 223.

Raghoebar GM, Schoen P, Meijer HJ, Stellingsma K, Vissink A. Early loading of endosseous implants in the augmented maxilla: a 1-year prospective study. Clin Oral Implants Res. 2003 Dec;14(6):697 – 702.

Rocci A, Martignoni M, Gottlow J. Immediate loading in the maxilla using flapless surgery, implants placed in predetermined positions, and prefabricated provisional restorations: a retrospective 3-year clinical study. Clin Implant Dent Relat Res. 2003;5 Suppl 1:29 – 36. (2006a)

Rocci A, Martignoni M, Gottlow J. Immediate loading of Brånemark system TiUnite and machined surface implants in the posterior mandible: a randomized open-ended clinical trial. Clin Implant Dent Relat Res. 2003;5 Suppl 1:57 – 63. (2006b)

Roccuzzo M, Bunino M, Prioglio F, Bianchi SD. Early loading of sandblasted and acid-etched (SLA) implants: a prospective split-mouth comparative study. Clin Oral Implants Res. 2001 Dec;12(6):572 – 8.

Roccuzzo M, Wilson T. A prospective study evaluating a protocol for 6 weeks' loading of SLA implants in the posterior maxilla: one-year results. Clin Oral Implants Res. 2002 Oct;13(5):502 – 7.

Romeo E, Chiapasco M, Ghisolfi M, Vogel G. Long-term clinical effectiveness of oral implants in the treatment of partial edentulism. Seven-year life table analysis of a prospective study with ITI dental implants system used for single-tooth restorations. Clin Oral Implants Res. 2002 Apr;13(2):133 – 43.

Romeo E, Lops D, Amorfini L, Chiapasco M, Ghisolfi M, Vogel G. Clinical and radiographic evaluation of small-diameter (3.3-mm) implants followed for 1 – 7 years: a longitudinal study. Clin Oral Implants Res. 2006 Apr; 17(2): 139 – 48.

Salama H, Rose LF, Betts NJ. Immediate loading of bilaterally splinted titanium root-form implants in fixed prosthodontics—a technique reexamined: two case reports. Int J Periodontics Restorative Dent. 1995 Aug;15(4):344 – 61.

Schatzker J, Horne JG, Sumner-Smith G. The effect of movement on the holding power of screws in bone. Clin Orthop Relat Res. 1975 Sep;(111):257 – 62.

Schincaglia GP, Marzola R, Scapoli C, Scotti R. Immediate loading of dental implants supporting fixed partial dentures in the posterior mandible: a randomized controlled split-mouth study—machined versus titanium oxide implant surface. Int J Oral Maxillofac Implants. 2007 Jan-Feb;22(1):35 – 46.

Schnitman P, Wohrle PS, Rubenstein JE. Immediate fixed interim prosthesis supported by two-stage threaded implants: methodology and results. Int J Oral Maxillofac Implants. 1997 Jul-Aug;12(4):495 – 503.

Schroeder A, Pohler O, Sutter F. Gewebereaktion auf ein Titan-Hohlzylinderimplantat mit Titan-Spritzschichtoberfläche. [Tissue reaction to an implant of a titanium hollow cylinder with a titanium surface spray layer.] SSO Schweiz Monatsschr Zahnheilkd. 1976 Jul;86(7):713 – 27.

Schwartz-Arad D, Laviv A, Levin L. Survival of immediately provisionalized dental implants placed immediately into fresh extraction sockets. J Periodontol. 2007 Feb;78(2):219 – 23.

Small PN, Tarnow DP. Gingival recession around implants: a 1-year prospective study. Int J Oral Maxillofac Implants. 2000 Jul-Aug;15(4):527 – 32.

Smithloff M, Fritz ME. The use of blade implants in a selected population of partially edentulous adults: A five-year report. J Periodontol. 1976 Jan;47(1):19 – 24.

Smithloff M, Fritz ME. The use of blade implants in a selected population of partially edentulous adults. A 15-year report. J Periodontol. 1987 Sep;58(9):589 – 93.

Soballe K, Hansen ES, B-Rasmussen H, Jorgensen PH, Bunger C. Tissue ingrowth into titanium and hydroxyapatite-coated implants during stable and unstable mechanical conditions. J Orthop Res. 1992 Mar;10(2):285 – 99.

Szmukler-Moncler S. Salama H, Reingewirtz Y, Dubruille JH. Timing of loading and effect of micromotion on bone-dental implant interface: review of experimental literature. J Biomed Mater Res. 1998 Summer;43(2):192 – 203.

Szmucler-Moncler S, Piattelli A, Favero G.A., Dubruille JH. Considerations preliminary to the application of early and immediate loading protocols in dental implantology. Clin Oral Implants Res. 2000 Feb;11(1):12 – 25.

Tarnow DP, Emtiaz S, Classi A. Immediate loading of threaded implants at stage 1 surgery in edentulous arches: ten consecutive case reports with 1- to 5-year data. Int J Oral Maxillofac Implants. 1997 May-Jun;12(3):319 – 24.

Tawse-Smith A, Payne AG, Kumara R, Thomson WM. Early loading on unsplinted implants supporting mandibular overdentures using a one-stage operative procedure with two different implant systems: a 2-year report. Clin Implant Dent Relat Res. 2002;4(1):33 – 42.

Testori T, Del Fabbro M, Feldman S, et al. A multicenter prospective evaluation of 2-month loaded Osseotite implants placed in the posterior jaws: 3-year follow-up results. Clin Oral Implants Res. 2002 Apr;13(2):154 – 61.

Testori T, Del Fabbro M, Szmukler-Moncler S, Francetti L, Weinstein RL. Immediate occlusal loading of Osseotite implants in the completely edentulous mandible. Int J Oral Maxillofac Implants. 2003 Jul-Aug;18(4):544 – 51.

Trisi P, Rao W. Bone classification: clinical-histomorphometric comparison. Clin Oral Implants Res. 1999 Feb;10(1):1 – 7.

Türkyılmaz I. A 3-year prospective clinical and radiologic analysis of early loaded maxillary dental implants supporting single-tooth crowns. Int J Prosthodont. 2006 Jul-Aug;19(4):389 – 90.

Türkyılmaz I, Sennerby, Tümer C, Yenigül M, Avcı M. Stability and marginal bone level measurements of unsplinted implants used for mandibular overdentures: a 1-year randomized prospective clinical study comparing early and conventional loading protocols. Clin Oral Implants Res. 2006 Oct;17(5):501-5. Click here to read

Vailati F, Belser UC: Replacing four missing maxillary incisors with regular- or narrow-neck implants: analysis of treatment options. Eur J Esthet Dent;2007;2:42 – 57.

Wiskott HW, Pavone AF, Scherrer SS, Renevey RR, Belser UC. Resistance of ITI implant connectors to multivectorial fatigue load application. Int J Prosthodont. 2004;17:672 – 679.

Wolfinger GJ, Balshi TJ, Rangert B. Immediate functional loading of Brånemark system implants in edentulous mandibles: clinical report of the results of developmental and simplified protocols. Int J Oral Maxillofac Implants. 2003 Mar-Apr;18(2):250 – 7.

Zarone F, Sorrentino R, Vaccaro F, Russo S. Prosthetic treatment of maxillary lateral incisor agenesis with osseointegrated implants: a 24-39-month prospective clinical study. Clin Oral Implants Res. 2006 Feb; 17(1): 94 – 101.

Zinsli B, Sagesser T, Mericske E, Mericske-Stern R. Clinical evaluation of small-diameter ITI implants: a prospective study. Int J Oral Maxillofac Implants. 2004 Jan – Feb; 19(1): 92 – 9.